The Quadruple Aim
in Nursing and Healthcare

T0197959

The Quadruple Aim in Nursing and Healthcare

*Improving Care, Lowering Costs,
Serving Populations,
Elevating Work Life*

SUE JOHNSON, PhD, RN, FAAN

McFarland & Company, Inc., Publishers
Jefferson, North Carolina

LIBRARY OF CONGRESS CATALOGUING-IN-PUBLICATION DATA

Names: Johnson, Sue (Carol Susan), 1946– author.
Title: The quadruple aim in nursing and healthcare : improving care, lowering
    costs, serving populations, elevating work life / Sue Johnson.
Description: Jefferson, North Carolina : McFarland & Company, Inc., Publishers,
    2020 | Includes bibliographical references and index.
Identifiers: LCCN 2020016606 | ISBN 9781476681085 (paperback) ∞
    ISBN 9781476640624 (epub)
Subjects: MESH: Institute for Healthcare Improvement. | Nursing Services—
    trends | Health Care Reform | Nursing—trends | Quality of Health Care |
    Nursing Care—organization & administration
Classification: LCC RT89 | NLM WY 105 | DDC 362.17/3—dc23
LC record available at https://lccn.loc.gov/2020016606

BRITISH LIBRARY CATALOGUING DATA ARE AVAILABLE

ISBN (print) 978-1-4766-8108-5
ISBN (ebook) 978-1-4766-4062-4

Front cover photograph by Billion Photos/LightField Studios

Printed in the United States of America

McFarland & Company, Inc., Publishers
    Box 611, Jefferson, North Carolina 28640
    www.mcfarlandpub.com

Acknowledgments

I wish to thank everyone who has contributed their ideas and comments that illustrate how current practice will impact healthcare in 2020 and beyond.

Special thanks to Beth Roszatkcki, CEO of Michigan Health Improvement Alliance, Inc. and Bill Baberg, President of InsightFormation Inc. for their insights about implementing the Quadruple Aim.

Table of Contents

Preface

"All great successes are the triumph of persistence."—
Ralph Waldo Emerson

Even today, 200 years after the birth of Florence Nightingale, the founder of modern nursing, her great success in multiple endeavors continues in the diverse roles of nurse leaders. Nursing has been recognized as the most trusted profession for the past 17 consecutive years according to Gallup's annual poll (National Nurses United, 2018). Trust carries responsibility to act in the best interest of patients, families, communities, and population health by nurses in multiple roles and settings. Although healthcare and nursing as a profession have changed significantly since Nightingale's time, her example aligns with current strategies to advance both.

Healthcare in the United States is a topic of national interest and discussion. There are multiple suggestions to reform and improve our healthcare system, but no one solution. This narrative is designed to explore the history of healthcare from Nightingale's time to the present and introduce the reader to the best available option to address the issues of our current and future healthcare system—the Institute for Healthcare Improvement's Quadruple Aim framework.

While the work of the non-profit Institute for Healthcare Improvement is not nursing specific, its Triple Aim framework for optimizing health system performance (Institute for Healthcare Improvement, 2018) is coherent with the nursing profession today. Furthermore, it has evolved to the Quadruple Aim, adding the improvement of provider work life (team vitality) to the original three: improved population health, improved experience of care for individuals, and lower costs. The future of healthcare depends on adoption of this framework nationally.

Governmental agencies and national organizations pursue the Quadruple Aim to address quality and cost issues in provision of healthcare in the United States. The National Quality Forum supports and safeguards the protection of patient populations and healthcare quality via measurement and public reporting. The National Quality Strategy uses a three-pronged approach—healthy people, better care, and affordable care—to improve health and healthcare quality for individuals and the community in which they live. This initiative is supported by Healthy People 2020, a framework developed in 1979 through collaboration of the Department of Health and Human Services (HHS), other federal agencies, public stakeholders, and an Advisory Committee on National Health Promotion and Disease Prevention composed of national public health experts. Healthy People 2020 establishes a 10-year plan to improve the well-being and health of people in the United States. The national, non-profit Leapfrog Group surveys U.S. hospitals on patient safety and quality measures and publicly reports results so individuals can select the highest quality care. HHS is the federal agency responsible for promoting affordable healthcare in the United States and has three divisions—CMS, AHRQ, and FDA—which are responsible for government-sponsored programs providing affordable care at the best cost.

In addition to these government and national groups, regional coalitions focus on achieving the Quadruple Aim with multiple activities designed to improve the health and well-being of individuals and populations in their communities using cost effective approaches. The work of one of these organizations—the Michigan Health Improvement Alliance (MiHIA)—is extensively profiled in this narrative. Such groups are vital to the success of the Quadruple Aim framework in communities throughout the United States. By involving stakeholders at all levels, supporting clinicians, and communicating effectively with residents, they are making a positive difference in their regions.

Nurse leaders are also vital to the achievement of these measures, and Nightingale's accomplishments lighted the way to their professional success today. The American Nurses Association and healthcare institutions nationwide support the physical, emotional, and social health of nurses and other healthcare team members with approaches such as resilience and mindfulness. Without a healthy team providing care, the recipients will not achieve an optimum level of health and well-being.

The personal and professional perceptions of 31 current nurse leaders in their own words are powerful statements about their commitment to the success of the Quadruple Aim framework to advance healthcare. These nurse leaders represent different sexes, generations, geographic areas, backgrounds, clinical, educational, and administrative expertise, and diverse positions in healthcare leadership. Their words are impactful along with their philosophy and vision for the nursing profession and healthcare in the United States. They are representatives of their peers and colleagues and their voice is essential to dialog about future healthcare delivery and changes. The reader will enjoy getting to know these nurse leaders within the narrative.

The future of healthcare is unknown, but Nightingale's triumph will be the impact of her nursing legacy on all aspects of care delivery, and numerous agencies, organizations, teams and individuals will use these skills to create affordable, high quality healthcare in the future. Individual and at-risk populations deserve no less.

This book is dedicated to the nurses and organizations profiled here; all the colleagues who have informed my practice over many years; our future nurse leaders; and Florence Nightingale, our mentor and guide to professional practice.

Happy 200th birthday, Florence!

Introduction

"Our vocation is a difficult one, as you, I am sure know; and though there are many consolations and very high ones, the disappointments are so numerous that we require all our faith and trust. But that is enough. I have never repented nor looked back, not for one moment."— Florence Nightingale (Cook, 1913a, pp. 137–138)

This book—published almost exactly on the 200th birthday of Florence Nightingale—has been a labor of love inspired, as is so much of modern nursing, by her massive contributions. The leaders quoted throughout the book span different generations, sexes, educational backgrounds, and multiple roles throughout the United States. Each is unique and was selected to share their varied perspectives about each of the IHI Quadruple Aim measures. They live Nightingale's vision daily in their professional and personal lives.

Why these measures and not others, and how are they an apt reflection on Nightingale's legacy to nurses and nursing? Improving the individual's experience of care through practice and education began with Nightingale's work in the Crimea and continues today where nurse leaders use Nightingale's patient focus daily to improve individuals' experience in multiple healthcare settings. As Nightingale sought to improve the health of at-risk populations, today's nurse leaders devote their energies to advance health for new and challenging at-risk populations. Reducing healthcare costs was less intense in Nightingale's time, although she succeeded in doing this in her first leadership position in London and again in the Crimea where she monitored supply costs to ensure that soldiers received essential provisions. Today's nurse leaders demonstrate accountability and responsibility for ensuring productivity and cost reduction in a rapidly changing healthcare environment. Improving provider work life (team vitality) was an important consideration to Nightingale as she advocated for nurses throughout her career. Today's nurse leaders also focus on the satisfaction of team members, noting that this results in reduced turnover and improved patient/client satisfaction.

Each nurse leader willingly revealed their innermost feelings about the profession they love. I am humbled to read their responses and proud to call them colleagues. Nightingale's triumph is their vast success. I know she would be impressed by how far nursing has come and realize that nurse leaders will continue to advance the profession and healthcare in the future to truly achieve the Quadruple Aim.

1

Nightingale's View
of Nursing's Future

> "...How deep is my interest, how intense my feeling for you and your work I need not tell you; every woman must feel the same. You have done a noble deed in beginning. God will grant you success."—Florence Nightingale to Ella Pirrie, a Belfast nurse, 14 October 1885 (Dossey, 2000, p. 377)

The year 1897 was the year of Queen Victoria's Diamond Jubilee. As part of the celebration, a Victorian Era Exhibition was developed with one section devoted to nursing. Florence Nightingale was 77 at the time and was requested to provide "photographs, busts, autographs and 'relics of the Crimean War'" (Cook, 1913b, p. 409). At first, she resisted the request, but was ultimately persuaded to send a bust of herself and an old carriage that she had used in the war. Privately, she considered these items frivolous and used the Exhibition to give thanks to God while viewing her role in the Crimea critically and praising the results of nursing since then. "How inefficient I was in the Crimea! Yet He has raised up Trained Nursing from it!" (Cook, 1913b, p. 410).

Nursing had indeed come a long way in the years since the Crimean War and Nightingale realized that she had established "a new art, and a new science" (Cook, 1913b, p. 365). Nursing was no longer the realm of drunks and prostitutes. It was a respected role for gentlewomen who were educated at the Nightingale School and other schools to provide care for the sick. Forty years of work by Florence Nightingale had positively changed public perception of nurses and that continues today.

Improving the Experience of Care for Individuals Through Education

From her earliest experiences in healthcare to her old age, Nightingale's primary focus was the patient. Hospitals in the mid–19th century

7

were dens of infection rather than places of healing. Besides recommending sanitary measures—cleanliness, hand hygiene, ventilation, and reduction of overcrowding—she advocated nursing assessment by careful observation of patients. In her own words: "In dwelling upon the vital importance of *sound* observation, it must never be lost sight of what observation is for. It is not for the sake of piling up miscellaneous information or curious facts, but for the sake of saving life and increasing health and comfort" (Nightingale, 1992, p. 70). She knew that nurses could not accurately observe and assess patients without training (education) and money from the Nightingale Fund (established to recognize her service in the Crimean War), which provided funding for the first Training School for Nurses in England in 1860. The Nightingale School was established at St. Thomas' Hospital based on an agreement that the hospital would provide facilities for the nurses' training and the Nightingale Fund would provide the cost of the training, including the payment of the probationers. Although Nightingale wasn't well enough to become superintendent, she selected Mrs. Wardroper as Matron and Mrs. Wardroper remained in the role for 27 years. Their collaboration ensured that Nightingale nurses were employed in hospitals and other public institutions and that these graduates received superb technical training and displayed the discipline to lead nursing in multiple locations throughout the world (Cook, 1913a).

Nightingale's experiment in trained nursing was repeated by her graduates, many of whom became Lady Superintendents and changed the face of nursing and healthcare worldwide. In the United States, Alice Fisher of Blockley Hospital in Philadelphia was a Nightingale nurse and Linda Richards of Massachusetts General Hospital in Boston completed her post-graduate work in England under Nightingale's direction. These women spread Nightingale's concepts in the United States where trained nurses were largely unknown (Cook, 1913a). Richards' contribution to the fledgling nursing profession was considerable. She first completed a nurse training program at the New England Hospital for Women and Children in October 1873 and was employed as Superintendent of the Boston Training School for Nurses from 1874 to 1876. Her tenure changed the perception of nurses as ignorant servants by requiring "class instruction as a regular part of the nurses' education" (L. Richards, Massachusetts General Hospital and the Massachusetts General Hospital Nurses' Alumnae Association, 2011, pp. 36–37). Although she had elevated nursing practice in the United States, Richards spent several months in England in 1877 studying under Nightingale and later served five years as a medical missionary in Kyoto, Japan, where she founded the first school of nursing in that country. Her accomplishments led to leadership roles at home culminating in her selection as "first president of the American Society of Superintendents of Training Schools for nurses" (Massachusetts General Hospital and Massachusetts General Hospital Nurses' Alumnae Association, 2011, p. 38).

American nurses' education was evolving and resulted in improved patient care based on the concepts of Florence Nightingale and adherence by nurse leaders and educators like Linda Richards and Adelaide Nutting, who left Canada to study nursing at Johns Hopkins Training School for Nurses in Baltimore in 1889. Mary Adelaide Nutting began her role in nursing education in 1894 when she became the Superintendent of Nurses and Principal of the Training School at Johns Hopkins. She focused on establishing a three-year nurse training program and used research and statistical analysis to determine the benefit of an eight-hour day for students with the third year dedicated to education about administration because "less work, more education is needed" (Marshall, 1972, p. 72). Eleven years later, she became the Chair of Hospital Administration at Teachers College (Columbia University). Before she left Johns Hopkins for New York City, Nutting addressed the 1906 Johns Hopkins graduating class and expressed her philosophy about the future of nursing education. "We are in urgent need of nursing schools founded on a separate and independent basis in which the course of study and training will be complete, each hospital contributing what it fairly can as a field for teaching and receiving of the student, what she must necessarily give in obtaining her practical training and experience. The formation of such a school is the next step forward" (Marshall, 1972, p. 138). In 1907, Adelaide Nutting had a brief visit in London with Florence Nightingale about the progress of American nursing. Both women came away from their encounter refreshed and Nutting returned to the United States to become the first nurse to attain professional rank in any university. Her tenure at Teachers College resulted in development of bachelor's and master's degrees and active faculty engagement in research. She wrote: "The education of nurses passes over into a new era. It is because for the first time in history the education of nurses is accorded the status and powers which are recognized in the conduct and development of other forms of professional education" (Marshall, 1972, p. 287).

While nurse leaders and educators like Linda Richards and Adelaide Nutting were advancing educational opportunities for American nurses, other nurses were focusing their efforts on excellent patient care. One of these nurses was Mary Eliza Mahoney who had the distinction of being America's first trained African American nurse. Mahoney became an untrained practical nurse at 18 and spent the next 15 years in the hospital in Roxbury where she supplemented her income by working as a cook, janitor, and washerwoman (Campbell, 2012). In 1878, she finally enrolled in the 16-month nursing program at the New England Hospital for Women and Children. Students were required to work 16-hour days caring for six patients, attend long lectures, and study during their minimal time off. Mary Eliza Mahoney was one of only four graduates and on August 1, 1879, became the first African American woman to attain her nursing license. Since hospitals did not hire staff nurses at that time, she registered with the Nurses Directory and did private duty nursing throughout the East Coast for about 30 years. Her reputation for excellence in patient care led to a stellar career where her clinical skills were in high demand. She also became a role model for other African American women who sought careers in nursing (Campbell, 2012; Davis, 1999). Although her time was occupied with her patients and her church, Mahoney advocated for racial equality in the nursing profession and supported women's suffrage (Darraj, 2005; Davis, 1999). Families who employed her were impressed by her professionalism and her dedication to her patients illustrated the words of Florence Nightingale: "The work that tells is the work of the skillful hand, directed by the cool head, and inspired by the loving heart" (Cook, 1913b, p. 384). Although respected by her colleagues, Mary Eliza Mahoney wasn't recognized until after her death. Today, the American Nurses Association presents the Mary Eliza Mahoney Award at each biennial convention to recognize a person who has demonstrated outstanding contributions to equal opportunities for minorities in nursing (Carnegie, 1991). She has posthumously received numerous awards and honors, including induction into the ANA Hall of Fame. However, she would be proudest of two community honors: renaming of the Roxbury Area 2 Family Life Center to the Mary Eliza Mahoney Family Life Center and a center established in her memory by the Community Health Project in Oklahoma that is dedicated to health services provision in isolated communities (Carnegie, 1991).

These early nursing pioneers knew that education was essential to improve the patients' care experience and the health of populations. As they were moving American nursing forward, Florence Nightingale was constantly improving education at the Nightingale School. When one of her graduates, Elizabeth Torrance, was appointed as Matron at the new Highgate Infirmary in 1869, nine Nightingale nurses reported to her. She collaborated with Nightingale and established a training school for nurses at Highgate. The nurses greatly impressed the Medical Superintendent there who wrote to Nightingale, "I have never seen such nurses; they are so thoroughly conversant with disease that one feels quite on one's mettle in practice. What strikes me most is the real interest they take in the work, and this is the secret of their success" (Cook, 1913b, p. 193). It was a fitting tribute to the quality of education and practice by Nightingale nurses.

Improving the Health of Populations

Nightingale also devoted much of her life to improving the health of populations. Her advocacy began in the Crimea where lack of basic supplies endangered the health and welfare of soldiers in the Scutari hospitals. She used her own supplies and collaborated with the three Sanitary Commissioners dispatched to the war zone to improve conditions for the soldiers there. Their focus on sanitation improved cleanliness, drainage, and ventilation as well as reducing overcrowding in the wards (Cook, 1913a). Nightingale used these principles during her lifetime to improve the health of multiple populations throughout the world. It was her first experience with Commissions, but far from the last. In 1862, she analyzed life in India, and her insights and "'Observations by Miss Nightingale,' which occupy twenty-three pages of the (Indian Sanitary Commission's) Report, are among the most remarkable of her Works, and in their results among the most beneficent. They are also extremely readable" (Cook, 1913b, p. 25). This paper circulated widely in England with even the Queen receiving a copy. Her advocacy for proper sanitation resulted in the establishment of a Sanitary Committee at the India Office in 1867 and subsequent appointment of local medical officers of health there. The health of the Indian population was a lifelong passion for Florence Nightingale. She realized that sanitary education was vital to the health of villagers throughout India and supported the entry of Health Missioners there to provide such education (Cook, 1913b).

Nightingale also passionately focused on the use of Health Missioners in England when she determined that education on sanitation was essential in rural villages there. She had support from one of the county councils who could levy and spend money on technical education. In 1890, more funds were available and technical education was broadly defined. Nightingale convinced the "chairman of the Technical Education Committee of North Bucks" (Cook, 1913b, p. 383) to use some of this money to provide practical sanitary education to housewives in the villages there. She believed that one-to-one instruction was the best approach for success. In 1892, Nightingale enlisted the help of the district Health Officer, a local physician. He taught the women volunteers practical and theoretical information about rural hygiene through classes and lectures. Then, he took his pupils to area villages, introduced them to women there, and created opportunities for them to help villagers by sharing knowledge about sanitary practices. At Nightingale's request, the students took an independent examination and those who passed served a probationary period before receiving certificates as Health Missioners. This approach to sanitary education improved the health of this rural population and Florence Nightingale's contribution was essential to its success. She recruited women for the program, provided information about best practices in sanitary education, developed syllabi and examinations, communicated with other technical education committees, and wrote papers and letters about rural hygiene. Her involvement in the Health Missioner program contributed largely to its success and made a positive difference in life in these rural villages (Cook, 1913b).

Nurses in the United States also focused on improving the health of populations through education. Lillian Wald's compassion for her patients extended to her community. After graduating in 1891, she tried to initiate reforms for children as a nurse at the New York Juvenile Asylum and left in frustration after a year (Williams, 1948). She enrolled in the women's Medical College of the New York Infirmary, but medicine didn't meet her needs. Her life changed when she taught a nursing class on Henry Street, an area of tenements and slums in New York City. Initially, Wald taught mothers in the area how to prepare nourishing meals and clean their households. When a little girl ran into her class asking help for her mother, Wald went with her to a squalid room where she found the mother bleeding after childbirth. She cared for her and cleaned the room. When she left, Lillian Wald knew what she wanted to do with her life (Williams, 1948; Block, 1969). The population of New York's Lower East Side contained poor immigrants from Germany, Italy and Ireland, and it also contained Eastern European Jews. Housing was poor with high rents and even poorly paid jobs were difficult to find. Many immigrants didn't speak English and were afraid of hospitals and visiting nurses (Block, 1969). Lillian Wald spoke with Betty Loeb, the philanthropist who financed the Henry Street class, and her son-in-law, Jacob Schiff, about providing funds for Wald and another nurse, Mary Brewster, to live in the neighborhood and gain the trust of its residents. They agreed and provided funds for medicines, medical supplies, and food for the sick (Williams, 1948).

The two nurses focused on building relationships with their neighbors. Following Nightingale's focus on cleanliness (Cook, 1913a; Cook, 1913b), they visited apartments, bathed and treated children, and taught mothers about cleanliness. They made janitors accountable for the condition of the buildings and convinced the Board of Health to sanction their work as visiting nurses (Block, 1969). Becoming a force in the community, Wald began the first public health nursing service to improve the residents' health and lives. Wald would have been surprised to learn that Florence Nightingale had foreseen this in 1876. In a letter to the *Times* in 1876, Nightingale wrote that nurses caring for the poor in their homes must have "a real home, within reach of their work, for the nurses to live in" (Cook, 1913b, p. 253). She also said that public health nursing was "twenty years ago a paradox, but twenty years hence will be a commonplace" (Cook, 1913b, p. 253). Lillian Wald would prove this during her career.

When Mary Brewster became ill and retired, Wald carried on. She moved to 265 Henry Street, where she attracted numerous nurses and other volunteers during the next 40 years. The many achievements of the Henry Street Settlement to population health included the first public playground, providing opportunities for children to read and play, the first school nursing program, development of special education classes for children with disabilities, child labor reform, and social clubs for all age groups (Block, 1969). Lillian Wald's experiment in public health nursing was replicated to improve population health around the world.

Another American pioneer in population health was also a nurse. Her name was Mary Breckinridge and her achievements resulted in the development of the Frontier Nursing Service in Kentucky (Breckinridge, 1952). Breckinridge was from a prominent Kentucky family. After serving as a volunteer nurse in France after World War I, she was determined to become a nurse-midwife. In 1922, Breckinridge spent time studying public health nursing at Teachers College of Columbia University. She studied nursing education, social sciences, statistics, public health, child and general psychology, and psychiatry (Breckinridge, 1952). She spent the summer of 1923 talking with midwives in Kentucky about their role and sailed to England that fall to study midwifery (Breckinridge, 1952). There she met Rosalind Paget, founder of the Midwives Institute, the first Queen's Nurse, and a Nightingale nurse. Among Breckinridge's prized possessions was a copy of *Introductory Notes on Organizing an Institution for Training Midwives and Midwifery Nurses* by Florence Nightingale. It was a gift from Adelaide Nutting at Teachers College. Paget recommended a four-month course for trained nurses at the Woolwich in London. Breckinridge enjoyed practicing district nursing there and became the first American certificated nurse-midwife. In 1924, Mary Breckinridge attained membership in the Midwives Institute (Breckinridge, 1952; Wilkie & Moseley, 1969).

When Mary Breckinridge returned home to Kentucky in 1925, she met with supporters, founded the Kentucky Committee for Mothers and Children, and started the first nurse-midwife service in three Kentucky counties. The death rate for American women in childbirth was the highest in the civilized world and almost 20,000 mothers and 200,000 infants died at birth or within one month post-delivery. There were more maternal deaths in the United States than deaths of Americans in all wars until that time. Plans were made for an annual audit, accurate records, free railroad passes for patients requiring transportation to the nearest city for hospital care, legal and professional status for nurse-midwives, arrangements for medical consultation, and location of services (Breckinridge, 1952; Wilkie & Moseley, 1969).

Breckinridge's attention to details and political savvy played a large role in the success of the Frontier Nursing Service (FNS). Nurses on horseback became a common sight in the Kentucky hills as Breckinridge hired nurse-midwives and public health nurses. She also believed that she and the other nurses must be neighbors of the population they served and established her home as the first local hospital as well as strategic nursing outposts in remote Kentucky locations. She used statistics and data to validate the contribution of the Frontier Nursing Service to these rural residents. That resulted in a health insurance plan by Metropolitan Life Insurance Company where home care and hospital services were available at a $1 annual fee with ability for patients to obtain services if they couldn't pay. This was one of the first managed health plans in the United States (Judd, Sitzman, & Davis, 2010).

Met Life conducted detailed studies of Frontier Nursing Services maternity cases at Breckinridge's request and Dr. Dublin of Met Life shared the findings and the impact on population health: "The study shows conclusively what has in fact been demonstrated before, that the type of service rendered by the Frontier Nurses safeguards the life of the mother and babe. If such a service were available to the women of the country generally, there would be 30,000 less stillbirths and 30,000 more children alive at the end of the first month of life. This study demonstrated that the first need today is to train a large body of nurse-midwives, competent to carry out the routines which have been established both in the FNS and in other places where good obstetrical care is available" (Breckinridge, 1952, p. 312).

Reducing Healthcare Costs

Florence Nightingale's experience with purveying (supply management) in the Crimea enabled her to advise the Army in June 1862 to remove the responsibility for controlling funds from the Commissariat and empower a separate Treasurer. "Would it not be better to have a separate Treasurer for the Army to receive all moneys and issue them to all departments? In private life nobody makes his steward or his butler his banker. It would not be economical. Finance is as much a specialty as marketing, and as much so, to say the least of it, in the Army as in private life" (Cook, 1913b, p. 64).

At Scutari, she noted that the transport system for medical supplies resulted in multiple sea voyages and that supplies had to be transported again after landing at additional expense. She advanced a solution to reform this system. "It is absolutely necessary that there should be a Government Store House, in the shape of a hulk, where stores for the British, from whatever ships, could be received at once from them, and be delivered on the ship-store-keeper's receipt. There are no store-houses to be had by the water's edge, and portage is very expensive and slow" (Cook, 1913a, p. 222).

In her first nursing leadership position as Superintendent at the Establishment for Gentlewomen during Illness at No. 1 Upper Harley Street in London, Nightingale reduced expenses per patient per day and convinced the General Committee there "that the successor to our House Surgeon (resigned) should be a dispenser, and dispense the medicines in the house, saving our bill at the druggist's of £150 per annum" (Cook, 1913a, p. 134). Another of her challenges there was the reluctance of the Committee and doctors to discharge patients who no longer met criteria for hospitalization. In these cases, Nightingale assumed that responsibility and her efficiency and cost effectiveness were lauded by the General Committee leaders (Cook, 1913a). This was a significant accomplishment in an era where men managed all finances.

In the United States, nurses were beginning to understand that efficiency and cost effectiveness required them to advance their practice in new arenas. One of these nurses was Annie Warburton Goodrich, whose myriad contributions to the profession and patient care reflected Nightingale's reliance on data analysis. Her focus on evidence began when she had a student rotation at Sloane Maternity Hospital. The medical superintendent complained that students didn't complete assignments in a timely fashion. Goodrich did a time study of this and found that the expectations of 11 hours of care actually took 17 hours! Although changes didn't occur as a result, she continued to focus on evidence (Koch, 1951). Her administrative skills grew at the New York Postgraduate Hospital where she collaborated with the Board to become superintendent of both nursing and the training school in a cost reduction initiative. For the next seven years, the program curriculum evolved, and the school met high standards and established collaborative relationships with physicians (Kock, 1951; Yost, 1955). During the next 10 years (1900–1910) Goodrich served as director and superintendent of training schools for St. Luke's Hospital, the New York Hospital, and Bellevue Hospital. Her focus on housekeeping issues on wards mirrored Florence Nightingale's at Harley Street and she also became interested in hospital design. Following Nightingale's example, she advocated for window placement for patients, planning for hospital expansion, availability of dumbwaiters or elevators, inclusion of closets for patients' clothing, and arrangements for heating and disinfection (Cook, 1913a; Yost, 1955). In 1910, Goodrich was appointed to a civil service position that enabled her to use data and reporting to recommend standards for nurses' training as Inspector of Nurses' Training Schools in New York State. Many schools provided inferior education or exploited their students. In 1912, 90 percent of women calling themselves nurses had no education or had only attended correspondence schools (Koch, 1951). Goodrich's review resulted in data used by the Superintendents' Society to promote legal requirements and establish standards for nurses' training (Yost, 1955).

Besides joining the faculty of Teachers College in 1914 and being elected president of the American Nurses Association in 1916, Goodrich became general director of the Henry Street Settlement and improved hours and salaries for the Settlement's nurses (Yost, 1955). Her reputation for comprehensive, data-driven review made her the logical candidate for Chief Inspecting Nurse of the Army Hospitals by the Surgeon General's Office in 1918 (Koch, 1951). Her evaluation of the quality of nursing services in military hospitals in the United States and abroad was unfavorable and resulted in her proposal to the Secretary of War in 1918 for an Army School of Nursing (Koch, 1951). Armed with his authorization, her proposal garnered support from the 24th annual convention of the National League of Nursing Education and a budget was approved in June 1918. The school was unique because it was a separate educational unit and contained an independent budget specifically for educational purposes (Donahue, 2011). With this budgetary resource, Goodrich became Dean of the Army School of Nursing, and in five months, 1,600 student nurses went to hospitals at 31 training camps with a director and staff of teachers and supervisors at each camp. Goodrich's nursing career continued beyond the war and the Army School of Nursing remained viable until 1931 (Koch, 1951). These achievements illustrate Annie Warburton Goodrich's judicious use of data and cost efficiency/effectiveness to support nurses and patients in diverse settings.

Another American nurse used her financial astuteness to create paths for minority African American nurses to succeed in the nursing profession. Mary Elizabeth Carnegie wanted an education but didn't have any money for college. After graduating from high school at 16, Elizabeth moved from Washington, D.C., to New York to seek education opportunities. She was accepted at the Lincoln School for Nurses, a school of nursing for blacks, by putting her age as 18 on her application (Houser & Player, 2007). After graduation, she worked in hospitals that hired black nurses and continued to pursue her own education. Attaining a bachelor's degree in sociology enabled Carnegie to teach nursing in the Black School at the Medical College of Virginia and subsequently to start the first BSN program in Virginia at Hampton University. After this she began a lasting relationship with the

Rockefeller Foundation that provided her with funding for a certificate of completion for nursing school administration at the University of Toronto. The Rockefeller Foundation then recommended Carnegie as the nursing dean at Florida A&M University where they were financing a new hospital on the condition that a nursing dean be in charge of the school of nursing. Later she asked the Foundation for another educational grant and attained a master's in education from Syracuse University. Her relationship with the Rockefeller Foundation was invaluable when she sought appropriate clinical sites for her students. Overcoming the prejudices of white nursing directors, Carnegie arranged with the Director of Nursing at Duval Medical Center in Jacksonville, Florida, for student clinicals there (Houser & Player, 2007). Then, she had clinical space, but no housing for her students. She convinced Florida A&M to request funding from the Rockefeller Foundation and these funds provided a house that accommodated 12 to 16 students. The grant funding "enabled the school to employ faculty members, a dietitian, a cook, office furniture for empty space within the hospital that had been set aside, a small library of books, and a furnished classroom" (Houser & Player, 2007, pp. 48–49).

Carnegie now had a clinical site, but she was determined that Florida A&M should have its own hospital on campus. She sought and received administration support and the Rockefeller Foundation came through again with a grant of $50,000 for construction. The school conducted a fund-raising campaign for the remainder of the funding, a few years later the groundbreaking occurred, and a modern new hospital was established (Houser & Player, 2007). Elizabeth Carnegie became a pioneer to numerous African American nurses and received many awards and accolades in her nursing career, and her relationship with the Rockefeller Foundation played a part in her success to open the nursing profession to black nurses.

Improvement of Provider Work Life (Team Vitality)

Team vitality was not a known concept in Nightingale's time, but she was aware that concern about families at home would affect the well-being and performance of her nurses in the Crimea. She had family and friends in England look out for her nurses' families, especially the children. Her sister, Lady Verney, said, "Many things turn up for us to do for Florence; as in looking after the children of her nurses" (Cook, 1913a, p. 198). Her mother, Mrs. Nightingale, put it this way: "Flo has been writing incessantly lately about her nurses' families, for whom the best seem getting very anxious, and she scarcely mentions anything else. We have seen and heard much in visiting them which is a great pleasure to us" (Cook, 1913a, p. 198).

Years later when graduates of the Nightingale School assumed responsible positions throughout the world, Florence Nightingale "was not only the queen of the Nightingale Nurses, she was also their mother. The principal lieutenants who went out on important service, and many members of the rank and file, maintained constant correspondence with her—sending to her direct reports, consulting her in difficulties, looking to her, and never in vain, for counsel and encouragement. Miss Nightingale took especial pains to help and to influence the Lady Superintendents who went from St. Thomas's in command of nursing parties" (Cook, 1913b, p. 191). Current nursing students also benefited from Florence Nightingale's attention. One of these students described a visit with her in this way: "She was always on the look-out to make your visit not only restful and restoring by all manner of material comfort, but to make it interesting and brightening as well" (Cook, 1913b, pp. 303–304).

In the United States, Lillian Wald's Henry Street Settlement became a positive place for nurses and other health team members to live and work. She trusted her staff to perform independently and praised their successes. It was a truly team approach to the care of their clients in the community. The team members demonstrated mutual respect, affection, and positive communication skills. One technique to reward her team members was Wald's use of handwritten notes congratulating them on a job well done. These notes contributed to team vitality and were treasured by her staff, who called them the "L.D.W. Degree" (Block, 1969, p. 113).

Two African American nurses also promoted team vitality among minority nurses and collaboration with leaders of other nursing organizations. Estelle Massey Riddle Osborne mentored Elizabeth Carnegie and was a national leader for African American nurses. She was a groundbreaker in many ways. After graduation and a Missouri State Board exam score of 93.3 percent, Estelle Massey spent three years as the first African American head nurse on a large hospital ward (Hine, 1989). After experiencing discrimination related to promotion opportunities, she taught for a while at the Lincoln School of Nursing in Kansas City. Realizing she needed more education, Massey resigned her instructor position and became the first recipient of the Rosenwald Fellowship for African American graduate nurses. She focused on her professional development and attained a BS in Nursing Education from Teachers College in 1930. A year later she became the first African American nurse with a master's degree in nursing education—making her the best-educated African American nurse in the United States (Hine, 1989; Mosley, 2004). New opportunities in nursing leadership beaconed and Massey took advantage of them. She became the Educational Director at Freedman's Hospital in Washington, D.C., now Howard University, and served on a team funded by the Rosenwald Foundation to study the health and welfare of African Americans in the South. Massey was becoming the best known African American nurse and she accepted an invitation from the Board of Directors at Homer G. Phillips Hospital, her alma mater, to become its first African American Director of Nursing (Mosley, 2004).

She married a physician named Riddle, but the marriage ended in divorce. Then Riddle devoted herself to her career and equality for African American nurses. She moved easily in and out of both integrated and segregated groups and developed strong relationships in the South and Midwest that were advantageous to her role as a social change agent (Hine, 1989). Riddle used these relationships to promote racial equality within the nursing profession.

Riddle became active in resurrecting the National Association of Colored Graduate Nurses (NACGN) in the 1930s. The organization had been inactive for years and had no clear mission or program. Membership was dwindling because African American nurses thought it was irrelevant to their practices and lives. Riddle became president in 1934 and served in that role for five years. Her focus was promoting membership and meeting with African American nurses throughout the United States to hear their ideas and concerns. Her approach revitalized NACGN into the premier organization for African American nurses. She also realized the importance of communication in developing team cohesiveness and created an information bureau for both African American nurses and the public (Hine, 1989). Riddle focused on education, professionalism, and practice opportunities for African American nurses, and her quiet diplomatic approach promoted negotiations with white nurse leaders and liaisons with philanthropists who supported and funded her efforts. Her commitment to cooperation resulted in her involvement in white nursing organizations as representative of African American nurses. She openly shared information to involve other African American nurses locally and in collaboration with other African American professional groups (Hine, 1989).

It was an uphill battle for social change and Riddle became a powerful spokesperson to improve educational opportunities for African American nurses when she became a consultant to the National Nursing Council for War Service in 1943. Her role as the first African American appointee was to work with professional organizations and politicians to eliminate discrimination in the Armed Services and white schools of nursing (Mosley, 2004). Timing was good because, in her own words, "pressure upon the over-all nursing supply helped to reduce racial barriers within the employment and educational areas of nursing" (Hine, 1989, p. 153). Her advocacy for African American nurses paid significant results over a two-year period. The number of nursing schools admitting them grew from 18 to 28 and the Army and Navy lifted bans on their service. The Cadet Nurse Corps enlisted 2,000 African American students and provided funds for their education (Mosley, 2004).

In 1945, she became the first African American nurse to join the NYU faculty and mentored African American students and nurses there. After her marriage to Herman Osborne in 1946, Estelle continued to provide leadership to improve race relations within the nursing profession and the country by establishing relationships within professional organizations (Hine, 1989; Mosley, 2004). In 1948, the American Nurses Association (ANA) was finally integrated. African American nurses became individual members and a resolution was adopted to establish biracial committees in state associations and districts to implement educational programs promoting intergroup relations. Osborne became the first African American nurse elected to the ANA Board of Directors (Hine, 1989).

Osborne had succeeded in her advocacy for racial equality in nursing and her quiet perseverance earned her respect and admiration throughout the profession. One of her greatest achievements was the creation of the Mary Eliza Mahoney Award in 1936 by NACGN to recognize outstanding achievement in "nursing and human service" (Hine, 1989, p. 126). When the NACGN merged with the American Nurses Association, ANA continued to present the award to "African American nurses who have demonstrated excellence in their field" (Darraj, 2005, p. 114). The 1946 Mary Eliza Mahoney Award went to an educator, administrator, advocate for racial equality in nursing, and social change agent—Estelle Massey Riddle Osborne.

Osborne's chief collaborator in NACGN and the movement for elimination of racial discrimination and professional integration of African American nurses was Mabel Keaton Staupers. She began her career as a private duty nurse. After a short marriage and divorce from Dr. James Max Keaton, Mabel returned to Harlem to work with two physicians at the first African American healthcare facility there, the Booker T. Washington Sanitarium. She was adept at community organizing, healthcare advocacy, and nursing administration as demonstrated by her work with Pennsylvania State Board officials on a project to standardize nurses' training (Hine, 1989). After additional education at the Pennsylvania School for Health and Social Work, Keaton assisted with a survey of health needs in Harlem and evaluated the services available to African Americans in both city and state tuberculosis facilities. Her survey was the rationale to establish the Harlem Committee of the New York Tuberculosis and Health Association and

Keaton became its first Executive Secretary. This visible position enabled Keaton to develop relationships with African American political and social leaders in New York City (Hine, 1989). Like Osborne in the Midwest and South, she developed a network of professional contacts in the Northeast.

Keaton used her organizational skills, humor, and energy to address tuberculosis-related issues (Hine, 1989). Her inclusive team approach resulted in health education lectures for the public, fresh-air summer camps for children, and health services providing free exams and dental care for schoolchildren. She also established prenatal clinics and advocated for the appointment of African American physicians to TB clinics and New York City hospitals. In 1931, she married Fritz Staupers of Barbados and continued her healthcare initiatives (Hine, 2004).

Staupers was integral in the revitalization of the NACGN and became its first salaried Executive Secretary in 1934. With support from the Rockefeller Foundation and the Julius Rosenwald Fund, the organization's office was located in Rockefeller Center in New York City (Hine, 2004). In that role, she traveled extensively meeting with nurses across the country and honestly sharing organization financial information with them. Her leadership helped African American nurses build coalitions with local African American leaders of organizations like the NAACP and the National Urban League. Then, Staupers encouraged organizing interracial citizens' committees across the United States. By 1942, there were 12 groups nationally whose purpose was improving the image of African American nurses and obtaining more employment opportunities for them in hospitals and visiting nurse services. She stated, "In doing this we are following the trend in other nursing organizations. This is valuable, since the nurse needs help and the layman needs to understand the nurse" (Hine, 1989, p. 126).

Besides creating permanent alliances with officers of several national African American organizations and the NACGN, Staupers expertly publicized the contributions of African American nurses to healthcare (Hine, 1989). When World War II began, she took on the challenge of integrating the Army and Navy Nurse Corps by creating an NACGN National Defense Committee to represent African American nurses across the United States. This committee's leaders met with the Surgeon General of the Army but didn't make progress toward integration in the armed services. Staupers then met with President Franklin Roosevelt who embraced nondiscrimination. However, the War Department sided with the Surgeon General's viewpoint that African American nurses could only be used if separate hospital facilities were required for African American troops (Hine, 1989).

Staupers mobilized the press and public support to criticize quotas for joining the Armed Forces Nurse Corps. She gained support from white nursing organizations and white philanthropists and was beloved by the African American public. Her visibility resulted in her appointment as the only woman on a subcommittee on Negro Health and under her leadership the NACGN supported an amendment to the legislation creating the Cadet Nurse Corps. This amendment ensured that African American student nurses could join the Corps (Hine, 1989). Progress was slow, but on January 20, 1945, the War Department ended the quotas and decreed that African American nurses could join the Navy Nurse Corps. Staupers' advocacy resulted in elimination of racial quotas and discrimination by the military. She also aligned multiple groups into cohesive coalitions to change laws and minds (Hine, 1989).

Staupers next cause was integrating African American nurses into the American Nurses Association. She and Osborne joined forces and in 1948 the ANA House of Delegates voted to accept African American nurses as individual members. Staupers' response was ecstatic: "The doors have been opened and the black nurses have been given a seat in the top councils. We are now a part of the great organization of nurses, the American Nurses Association" (Hine, 2004, p. 612). After this success, Staupers returned to the NACGN as president and guided the organization to dissolution because it had served its purpose.

In 1951, the Spingarn Committee of the NAACP awarded Staupers the prestigious Spingarn Medal with this statement: "You were willing to sacrifice organization to ideals when you advocated and succeeded in realizing full integration of Negro nurses into the organized ranks of the nursing profession of this country" (Hine, 1989, p. 186). Staupers' inclusive approach made African American nurses valued members of the healthcare team.

Summary

These examples illustrate how Nightingale and her successors in the United States improved the individual's experience of care through education, improved the health of at-risk populations, reduced healthcare costs, and fostered team vitality (improvement of provider work life). Unfortunately, these advances have not extended into all healthcare settings and are still challenges for many providers. Based on this historical perspective, what is happening in our current healthcare environment?

2

IHI's Triple (Now Quadruple) Aim Initiative

"We are only on the threshold of nursing. In the future, which I shall not see, for I am old, may a better way be opened! May the methods by which every infant, every human being, will have the best chance of health—the methods by which every sick person will have the best chance of recovery, be learned and practiced!"—Florence Nightingale (Dossey, 2000, p. 375)

Nightingale's quote was even more prophetic than she knew. Higher quality healthcare continues to be a prime objective in today's environment. The impetus began in 1987 when Donald M. Berwick, M.D., and A. Blanton Godfrey, chairman and CEO of Juran Institute, Inc., launched the National Demonstration Project in Quality Improvement in Health Care to evaluate if higher quality required higher costs. Twenty-one healthcare organizations participated in an eight-month study to determine if industrial quality improvement methods could be applied in healthcare. They were supported by 21 business organizations who provided free consultation, access to training courses, materials, and reviews. These business organizations included Ford, IBM, AT&T, Xerox, and Corning and represented many of the United States' leading quality corporations. After eight months, 15 of the healthcare organizations had substantial results resulting in a three-year extension (Godfrey, 1996).

The project demonstrated that use of quality improvement methods (e.g., flowcharts, fishbone diagrams, Pareto diagrams, histograms, run charts, and control charts) was effective in resolving healthcare problems. Each of the successful healthcare organizations used these methods to address issues specific to their facilities. These issues ranged from problems transferring appropriate emergency department data to satellite sites, reducing delays in ambulatory surgery, improving emergency services, meeting demands for respiratory care in a timely fashion, reducing billing delays and inaccuracies, improving emergency department processes and increasing laboratory response times (Berwick, Blanton, & Rossner, 1990).

Quality management professionals guided teams within each organization to diagnose the problem, identify the root causes of workflows in the process, and develop solution(s) for testing and implementation. The teams discovered ways to implement solutions successfully. These methods included encouraging participation by everyone, providing enough time to test and implement the solution, maintaining the focus of the project, collaborating closely with organization leaders, and avoiding blame by treating everyone with respect and dignity (Berwick, Blanton, & Rossner, 1990).

Organizations focused on removing processes that didn't function at optimum levels. For example, if phlebotomy equipment was difficult to use, investment in new supplies could result in long-term savings at minimal cost. Inspection was important to determine if the proposed solution was effective. Human errors were also addressed and changes in policies and procedures supported the proposed solutions. They discovered that improved communication and measurements among departments resulted in increased improvement opportunities. It was important to sustain the results by monitoring how well the solution improved processes and if the improvement was maintained over time (Berwick, Blanton, & Rossner, 1990).

Measurement of results and variables in the process was challenging. After clearly identifying what the new process should accomplish and setting clear performance targets, measurement was essential to evaluate actual performance, compare this performance to targets, and act when there were differences between expected performance and actual performance. Success wasn't measured by one project's achievements. It was the cumulative result of numerous projects over time and increased usage of quality improvement methodology within the organization. Success also reflected positive attitudes about this approach to solving problems. Sometimes, the improvement process could be transferred to another department. Other times, ideas that occurred in one project could be used in other departments. Cross-functional teams played a role in improving healthcare processes, and the support of organization leaders was vital to the success and utilization of quality improvement processes (Berwick, Blanton, & Rossner, 1990).

These are lessons learned from the National Demonstration Project on Quality Improvement in Health Care that led to the creation of the Institute for Healthcare Improvement, and, ultimately, the Quadruple Aim.

Mission, Vision and Values

In 1991, the project evolved into the Institute for Healthcare Improvement (IHI) which continues to be committed to the "science of improvement" (Institute for Healthcare Improvement [IHI], 2018). IHI is guided by its mission, vision and values; understanding them is essential to understanding the organization and its functions. The vision is worded simply but delineates a lofty future goal: "Everyone has the best care and health possible" (IHI, 2018). IHI's mission is designed to achieve this vision: "Improve health and healthcare worldwide" (IHI, 2018).

The organization's eight values are a blueprint for action and are integral to success.

1. People matter—IHI's staff believe in treating everyone with dignity and respect. They are aware that everyone involved in the process—staff members, faculty members, partner organizations, and healthcare workers—has knowledge and experience that contribute to innovative solutions. Interactions must be positive, respectful, and cooperative (IHI, 2018).

2. Boundarilessness—IHI is a cohesive team with shared knowledge and systems that is not limited by structural boundaries. They believe and practice that "all teach, all learn" (IHI, 2018).

3. Innovation and Systems Thinking—Every system if unchanged will continue to produce the same results. For IHI and its partner organizations to make a difference in health and healthcare quality worldwide, there must be "continuous innovation and improvement of systems" (IHI, 2018).

4. Equity, Diversity, and Inclusion—IHI endeavors to "have an organization that reflects the world we live in and embraces everyone in it, no matter where they come from, no matter what their point of view" (IHI, 2018).

5. Generosity—IHI shares its knowledge with others near and far to make a "significant and lasting impact" (IHI, 2018).

6. Transparency—IHI is truthful and openly shares failures along with successes "to accelerate the learning on how best to improve" (IHI, 2018).

7. Speed and Agility—IHI anticipates how its work will be impacted by rapid changes in healthcare so the organization can "respond as quickly as necessary to support the transformation of healthcare" (IHI, 2018).

8. Celebration and Thankfulness—The IHI workforce celebrates

successes and takes time to thank each other for their accomplishments (IHI, 2018).

The Science of Improvement

Using a scientific approach, IHI begins by defining a clear target for improvement and leveraging the expert knowledge of multiple professions to address measurement tools and methods for change (IHI, 2018). Their focus is beginning with small tests of change using the Plan, Do, Study, Act (PDSA) model developed by the Associates in Process Improvement following W. Edwards Deming's theory of improvement and management called the System of Profound Knowledge. Dr. Deming's system includes theories of systems, psychology, knowledge, and variation and reflects his belief that using his theory will help organizations increase quality while reducing costs (IHI, 2018).

Model for Improvement

The Associates in Process Improvement (API) consists of six national associates who conduct research and development activities, assist organizations in integrating Dr. Deming's system with their subject knowledge, and help lead collaborative improvements with all stakeholders. API's Plan, Do, Study Act (PDSA) model addresses three questions: "What are we trying to accomplish? How will we know that a change is an improvement? What change can we make that will result in improvement?" (Associates in Process Improvement [API], 2018).

API's principles are reflected in their relationships with clients, suppliers and associates.

1. API associates' shared knowledge is vital when interacting with clients. API provides ongoing development opportunities for their associates to increase their job satisfaction and enable them to deliver the best possible service to clients (Associates in Process Improvement, 2018).

2. API associates "focus on understanding the contributions of both the system and the individual" (Associates in Process Improvement, 2018).

3. API associates develop mutually beneficial long-term relationships based on trust with suppliers (Associates in Process Improvement, 2018).

4. API associates carefully monitor resource utilization for both API and their clients (Associates in Process Improvement, 2018).

5. All API associates use science of improvement methods and principles in their direct involvement "in leadership and running the business" (Associates in Process Improvement, 2018).

The Institute for Healthcare Improvement uses Associates in Process Improvement methodology to effect positive change that is cost effective and enhances quality. IHI's science of improvement begins with a clear improvement goal and a plan to measure results. After using the PDSA model to test changes on a small level, results are refined for implementation on a larger scale. Organizations can partner with IHI's dedicated Innovation Team "to research innovative ideas, assess their potential for advancing quality and safety in healthcare, and bring them to action" (IHI, 2018). This 90-Day Learning Cycle process identifies problems that hinder progress and delineates how the organization can use rapid cycle tests to implement a workable solution (IHI, 2018). The team scans literature and talks to key innovators and experts about the problem in the first 30 days. These may include experts outside healthcare who have valuable input. A charter for the project defines the goal to achieve and deliverables essential to success. At the end of 30 days, the team has "a description of the current environment, a set of prevailing theories and mental models about how others have approached the problem before and an annotated bibliography" (IHI, 2018).

Using these details and comprehensive requirements to develop an innovative solution, the next 30–45 days focuses on testing theories at the point of care and seeing how they work. The final 15–30 days confirms the theory and the team develops a final summary and synthesis to disseminate to a team for testing and/or implementation (IHI, 2018).

The Triple Aim

The Institute for Healthcare Improvement has become an influential voice in healthcare redesign in the years since 1991. Originally, IHI concentrated on identifying and diffusing best practices to reduce microsystem or unit-based errors. This evolved into innovative solutions to problems in hospital systems. Finally, IHI ascertained an approach to improve the healthcare system in the United States, called the Triple Aim (IHI, 2018). In 2008, the Institute for Healthcare Improvement under the direction of Donald Berwick, M.D., President & CEO, began pursuing interdependent goals of improving individuals' care experience, improving population health, and reducing per capita cost of healthcare (IHI, 2018). The organization realized that a systematic approach to change is essential at all levels of the healthcare system and conducted six phases of pilot testing with more than 100 organizations worldwide. Their resulting recommendation for the change process included "identification of target populations; definition of system aims and measures; development of a portfolio of project work that is sufficiently strong to move system-level results; and rapid testing and scale up that is adapted to local needs and conditions" (IHI, 2018). IHI believes that to ensure that every person's lifetime journey through the healthcare system is flawless, patients and families must be empowered, community health issues must be addressed, and primary care and other community-based services must be expanded (IHI, 2018).

In the past few years, progress has been made toward the Triple Aim. Progress includes new primary care models, such as patient-centered medical homes; advent of bundled payments for care of certain illnesses; implementation of accountable care organizations; financial sanctions for avoidable events (e.g., infections, hospital readmissions); and integration of information technology (IHI, 2018). Measures have been defined for each aspect of the Triple Aim, but concerns remain about achieving them. IHI's high level measures (e.g., remaining years of healthy life, potential years of life lost) are useful in developing long range plans. Data from Hospital Compare, Centers for Medicare and Medicaid Services (CMS), or some National Committee for Quality Assurance (NCQA) measures impact at a project level. IHI recommends that facilities and providers create the ability to use existing data for improvement. Delays in obtaining publicly reported data may be as long as a year. Although this data is less useful in improvement initiatives, its trends may compare with national or state results. It can also be supplemented by health plans' utilization data and Medicare data. Some measures would be useful at the local or county level but are aggregated only at the state level. It may be necessary to obtain data from local hospitals and businesses about the impact of health premium increases to per capita spending (IHI, 2018).

Progress Report on the Triple Aim

Some headway is being made, but Triple Aim outcomes are still a work in progress. Primary care is the gateway to improved population health and individual access to healthcare and preventive services. Excellent primary care improves population health and equity while reducing costs (Kravitz & Feldman, 2017).

New Primary Care Models

Historically, primary care has been provider-centric with the physician totally accountable for the delivery of services to individuals seeking care. As reimbursement systems evolved, many primary care physicians were confronted with constraints on time spent interacting with clients because of increased regulatory and administrative responsibilities required to keep the practice solvent. Physicians are frustrated with increased paperwork to qualify for reimbursement that restricts the time they can spend treating their patients (Doherty, Robert, for the Medical Practice and Quality Committee of the American College of Physicians, 2015).

Although many primary care practices are traditional third-party fee-for-service in payment structures that focus on the quantity of care provided, new primary care models are evolving that enable individuals to receive ongoing and preventive care by physicians of their choice. These new models include direct primary care, concierge care, and split practices. Direct primary care offers quality care at an affordable price for individuals who pay a monthly or periodic fee to the practice. The practice does not bill for any third-party payments and charges for each visit are less than the monthly amount of the fee (Eskew & Klink, 2015). The concierge model also charges a monthly or periodic fee that is generally larger and attracts more affluent individuals. Some concierge practices also bill third parties in traditional fee-for-service as well as charging the periodic fee. Other practices use a hybrid or split practice approach where some individuals are treated in the direct patient care model and others use the traditional fee-for-service model. Many physicians in direct patient care practices must opt out of Medicare reimbursement if they want to treat Medicare clients because Medicare regulations ban physicians from charging Medicare clients for primary care services using the direct patient care model (Eskew & Klink, 2015).

Individuals seek direct care practices because of increased availability and access to their doctors. Their physicians have more time to spend with them leading to better quality and lower overhead costs. Cost reduction results from decreased overhead by eliminating third-party billing. These direct care practices tend to be small independent practices with different levels of affiliation with networks; split practices that are either totally independent or solely dependent on a network for their patients; or larger practices that employ physicians and market themselves directly to large employers to spur growth. Most direct care practices are newer and small, but larger practices are growing at faster rates when large employers purchase their plans for employees. Direct patient care practices are located in both urban and rural settings. Wider adoption of this model will require additional data to validate how these practices improve care (Eskew & Klink, 2015).

The Agency for Healthcare Research and Quality (AHRQ) realizes that primary care is the gateway to healthcare and wants to facilitate quality improvement and practice redesign to improve healthcare in the country. The agency has created several tools to help primary care practices achieve this. The AHRQ Health Literacy Universal Precautions Toolkit is a resource to help individuals understand health information and is available for all literacy levels. Capacity building helps primary care practices build capacity for quality improvement and care coordination, helps organize patient care activities, and shares information by all of the healthcare team to provide safe, effective care to individuals. Clinical-community linkages help connect providers, public health agencies, and community groups to improve individuals' access to both "preventive and chronic care services" (AHRQ, 2018). Guide to Improving Patient Safety in Primary Care Settings by Engaging Patients and Families is a guide being created by AHRQ to help individuals, families, and primary care health professionals collaborate and promote care improvements. This project is ongoing and is creating approaches to increase patient safety by engaging individuals and their support network in primary care settings. Healthcare/system redesign makes "systematic changes to primary care practices and health systems to improve the quality, efficiency, and effectiveness of patient care" (AHRQ, 2018). Health information technology integration uses electronic approaches to manage healthcare information about individuals and populations to improve quality of care and cost effectiveness. Primary care practice–based research networks consist of collaboration by primary care practices and clinicians to address healthcare questions impacting the community and use evidence-based practice to advance health. Behavioral and mental health issues, including substance misuse, are commonly seen in primary care practices with co-morbidities and these providers are in a position to address these needs. Self-management support in primary care practices promotes "patient-centered care and care coordination" (AHRQ, 2018). AHRQ has created resources in the Prevention and Chronic Care program that primary care practitioners can use to apply self-management support (AHRQ, 2018).

Patient-Centered Medical Home

Another aspect of changes in primary care is the patient-centered medical home. In 2006, the American Academy of Family Physicians commenced the first National Demonstration Project (NDP) to examine a comprehensive patient-centered medical home model in a national sample of 36 family medicine practices across the United States. This NDP model was monitored over a two-year period. The model focused on implementing technology even though financial incentives and full technological availability were absent. A few practices succeeded in using technology while achieving positive patient perceptions of the patient-centered medical home. Interestingly, many other practices found lower patient satisfaction as they implemented these changes. It was challenging to keep the patient at the center of care in the patient-centered medical home. The results of using the NDP model showed that the patient experience, staff and clinician competencies, and use of technology must be intertwined to be successful (Crabtree, et al., 2010). As the patient-centered medical home gained recognition, AHRQ developed five characteristics that should be contained in these medical homes. These included (1) comprehensive care that uses a team-based approach to meet most of the "patient's physical and mental healthcare" (AHRQ.gov, 2018); (2) patient-centered care by including patients and families as care partners; (3) coordinated care that provides effective transitions across all care sites; (4) accessible services with minimal waiting, improved office hours, and better after-hours access to providers; and (5) quality and safety by "providing safe, high-quality care through clinical decision-support tools, evidence-based care, shared decision-making, performance measurement, and population health management" (AHRQ. gov, 2018).

The patient-centered medical home is a positive concept that can improve both primary care and care for individuals requiring chronic care because these individuals are partners in care delivery. Technology facilitates sharing of information and communication, so patients are equipped to participate in their own care. As this model evolves, primary care practices cannot shoulder the costs of transforming their practices. Capital funding must include support from federal, state, and local agencies, health systems, and insurers. Ultimately, reform of our health system will be essential to support the success of the patient-centered medical home throughout the United States (Crabtree, et al., 2010).

Accountable Care Organizations

Accountable Care Organizations (ACOs) are groups of healthcare providers who are responsible for the costs and care delivery for specific patient populations. These groups receive financial incentives when they meet cost and quality targets by concentrating on primary care, care coordination, and preventing medical errors in care delivery (Lewis, et al., 2014). ACOs developed from rules created in 2011 by Health and Human Services (HHS) to provide better care coordination under the Patient Protection and Affordable Care Act. Accountable Care Organizations obtain financial rewards to ensure that patient populations receive the correct care at the right time to avoid duplication of services and medical errors especially when treating chronically ill populations. These organizations have grown exponentially in the past several years and many have contracted with CMS to manage care of Medicare beneficiaries and with private payers (Phillips-Jones, 2018).

ACOs received bonuses initially when reporting quality metrics. In 2013, the CMS program moved to pay for performance. This Medicare Shared Savings Program (MSSP) compensates ACOs for reducing growth in healthcare costs while meeting performance standards for patient-centered care and quality in clinical practice. More than 200 ACOs are enrolled in MSSP under a contract to manage healthcare needs for at least 5,000 Medicare recipients for a minimum of three years using CMS quality measures (Phillips-Jones, 2018).

In addition to involvement in the Medicare program, ACOs are located in almost every state and many seek to form partnerships with providers, primary care practices, hospitals, and other healthcare organizations to attain mutual or congruent goals. These "partnership ACOs" benefit all participants by risk-sharing or resource allocation (Lewis, Tierney, Colla, & Shortell, 2017). ACOs select partners with resources or expertise they require, and providers seek to reduce actual or perceived financial risks, by keeping significant segments of care delivery in the network, improving utilization monitoring, and meeting quality and cost benchmarks. ACOs also must meet minimum patient numbers to leverage financial risks when managing specific patient populations. These partnership ACOs will impact the success of the ACO model as they gain traction in the healthcare environment. Small provider organizations can maintain better autonomy and control as they participate in value-based care and contribute to improved care coordination and population health with ACOs. The future of such partnerships is unknown and partnership ACOs may be a permanent healthcare model or a transition phase as more organizations consolidate in the future (Lewis, Tierney, Colla, & Shortell, 2017).

Improved data and analytics enable care to be evaluated on outcomes, and this is evident in current value-based care and reimbursement. Medicare ACOs have demonstrated small cost reductions since their inception. Medicare is developing models that will encourage ACOs to take innovative financial risks for greater rewards when managing population health. Partnership ACOs have achieved small cost savings to date and initially score lower than existing organizations on quality measures for preventive health and at-risk populations. For partnership ACOs to succeed, the partners must establish trust in data and each other. These organizations have the potential to increase collaboration that benefits them and the populations they serve. This will be essential as the United States moves to a clinically integrated, coordinated and value-based healthcare system in the future (Lewis, Tierney, Colla, & Shortell, 2017).

The Quadruple Aim

IHI did not add team vitality as the fourth aim but supports other organizations that believe it is essential to achieving their organizational strategy to accomplish the original Triple Aim. IHI's focus is improving people's lives. Their leaders understand that the original job is not done. Individuals must be at the center of care; the care experience must be improved; gaps in population health must be removed; resources must be deployed cost-effectively to ensure the success of the Triple Aim; and organizations must measure essential data rather than measuring multiple items that divert attention from what is truly important (IHI, 2018). IHI agrees that team vitality is a key strategy in achieving Triple Aim outcomes because work-related stress and burnout are hazards to a positive care experience for patients (IHI, 2018).

Where Did It Come From?

The Quadruple Aim framework evolved from a group of medical professionals supported by a grant from the American Board of Internal Medicine Foundation which made site visits to 23 high-performing primary care practices throughout the United States in 2011 and 2012. These sites included "small private practices, large integrated delivery systems, academic medical centers, the Veterans Affairs, and Federally Qualified Health Care Centers" (Sinsky, et al., 2013, p. 273). The site visits were triggered by reports of burnout and decreased interest in adult primary care by physicians. Results showed that teamwork, interaction, and standardized work flows improved the work environment in these practices. Shared responsibility among team members promoted continuity and efficiency. Increased clinical support staff members and open communication resulted "in high-functioning teams, improved professional satisfaction, and greater joy in practice" (Sinsky, et al., 2013, p. 277).

In 2014 this survey team extrapolated these results to IHI's Triple Aim. Clinicians in primary care practices visited by the team expressed the following concern: "We have adopted the Triple Aim as our framework, but the stressful work life of our clinicians and staff impacts our ability to achieve the three aims" (Bodenheimer & Sinsky, 2014, p. 573). This concern evolved into the fourth aim which they defined as "improving the work life of healthcare clinicians and staff" (Bodenheimer & Sinsky, 2014, p. 573). This emphasis on team vitality as essential to achieving Triple Aim outcomes is recognized as a key strategy by IHI. Derek Feeley, current IHI President and CEO, clarified this in his Line of Sight column in November 2017: "Feel free to interpret the Triple Aim in a way that makes sense for you and your organization and what you need to achieve, but do so in a way that is deliberate and strategic. Whether you choose to work on the Triple Aim or the Quadruple Aim, understand that you can't ignore joy in work or equity and expect to secure Triple Aim outcomes" (Feeley, 2017).

Improvement of Provider Work Life (Team Vitality)

The Institute for Healthcare Improvement has established a framework to improve joy in work. As they explored this topic, they discovered that significant literature exists on factors associated with joy at work and that operational process improvement tools can be applied to improve provider work life and team vitality. IHI conducted three 90-day Innovation Projects on this topic in 2015–2016 to design and test a framework for health systems to improve team vitality. Current literature about satisfaction, engagement, and burnout were reviewed and over 30 interviews were performed with patients and selected exemplary healthcare and other organizations to address findings from the literature review. Site visits provided additional data and 11 healthcare organizations and systems spent two months testing a model program, improving the framework, and identifying areas for improvement (Perlo, et al., 2017).

Why Is the Fourth Aim Important?

Burnout in healthcare workers results in increased turnover and decreased morale. It affects the financial strength of healthcare organizations and "leads to lower levels of staff engagement, which correlate with lower customer (patient) experience, lower productivity, and an increased risk of workplace accidents" (Perlo, et al., 2017, p. 5). Burnout is linked to reductions in quality patient-centered care and safety as providers focus on their own needs in stressful work environments. However, focusing only on the

2. IHI's Triple (Now Quadruple) Aim Initiative

negative aspects of burnout won't solve the problem. Focusing on positive aspects of joy in work and team vitality is an approach that can improve care by nurturing compassion, caring, and dedication of healthcare personnel (Perlo, et al., 2017).

Joy in work and team vitality are beyond the absence of burnout and connect healthcare personnel to the purpose and meaning of their roles. Leaders can use this approach to promote resilience and innovative solutions that prevent burnout and make work a more enjoyable experience. W. Edwards Deming's theory of improvement also centers on joy in work. Using a manufacturing context, Deming wrote in his book *Out of the Crisis* two points that address this topic: Point 11, "Remove barriers that rob the hourly worker of his right to pride of workmanship," and Point 12, "Remove barriers that rob people in management and engineering of their right to pride of workmanship" (Perlo, et al., 2017, p. 6). Deming believed that joy in work is a basic right and that "management's overall aim should be to create a system in which everybody may take joy in [their] work" (Perlo, et al., 2017, p. 6).

Fairness and equity contribute to joy in work by addressing discrimination to drive engagement by employees. Outcomes from emphasis on joy and team vitality include better engagement, improved satisfaction levels, more positive individual patient experience, reduced burnout, and decreased turnover rates. Research studies have confirmed the link between better engagement and improved team performance. This increases productivity and results in reduced turnover and lower costs related to improved outcomes, safety, and individual patient experience ratings (Perlo, et al., 2017).

How Can Leaders Promote Progress Toward the Fourth Aim?

There are four steps that leaders can use to promote team vitality and joy in work. The first is the foundation of the other three and consists of asking team members what matters to them at work. Leaders must realize that they are there to listen and learn, not to solve every problem. The Institute for Healthcare Improvement has developed a guide for leaders to use in these conversations. The second step is to identify processes and issues that hamper progress toward attainment of team vitality. The leader's job doesn't end with just discovering barriers to success in this aim. They must also act on these issues starting with small tests of improvements at the unit level. Delaying action creates frustration among team members who don't see evidence of change that addresses their challenges. The third step is to bring teams together in shared responsibility for success. A senior leader should champion these efforts when the scope is beyond the unit level. The fourth step is testing tactics to improve team vitality and joy in work by improvement science methodology (Perlo, et al., 2017).

These four steps will have different answers in different organizations. What matters to individuals and what hinders success at the unit level go hand in hand. Huddles, communication boards, and team meetings begin the process of priority setting to mutually address barriers. Leaders must realize that building and engaging teams is their job and that everyone in the organization has a role in team vitality. There are nine core elements that denote shared responsibility for "a happy, healthy, productive workforce" (Perlo, et al., 2017, p. 12). These elements are (1) physical and psychological safety; (2) meaning and purpose; (3) choice and autonomy; (4) recognition and rewards; (5) participative management; (6) camaraderie and teamwork; (7) daily improvement; (8) wellness and resilience; and (9) real-time measurement (Perlo, et al., 2017, p. 13).

Senior leaders are responsible for all nine elements. Managers and first-line leaders are responsible for elements 5–9 and individual employees are responsible for elements 7–9. IHI's Framework for Improving Joy in Work begins by addressing fairness and equity; physical and psychological safety; meaning and purpose; choice and autonomy; and camaraderie and teamwork. The Model for Improvement that was discussed earlier is an effective way of using improvement science and a systems approach to increase team vitality and joy in work. After establishing a clear aim that can be measured, it is important to start with small tests of change and use data to improve future testing. It's also a good idea to be sure the change works before going beyond small tests. Every test result is valuable, so team members can use the data to improve processes. The Model for Improvement involves everyone in the organization, not just leaders (Perlo, et al., 2017).

Each of the nine steps in IHI's Framework for Improving Joy in Work contributes to team vitality and engagement. Physiological and psychological safety creates a fair environment and just culture. Meaning and purpose connects individuals' daily work to the organization's mission, vision, and purpose. Choice and autonomy encourage flexibility at work. Recognition and rewards demonstrate appreciation by leaders of team members' work and celebrate outcomes. Participative management encourages leaders to communicate with and listen to team members when making decisions. Camaraderie and teamwork support trust and mutual understanding in productive work teams. Daily improvement involves seeking opportunities for improvement by learning from deficiencies and successes. Wellness and resilience promote self-care, stress management, and work/life balance.

Real-time measurement involves regular feedback and honest assessments (Perlo, et al., 2017).

Team vitality and joy in work must be a key organizational priority and measured as all other priorities are measured. It is positively linked to patient experience, population health, and reduced costs from turnover and low employee morale. The fourth aim impacts the other three and deserves consideration for all to succeed.

3

Today's Nurse Leaders and the Quadruple Aim

"The thoughts and feelings that I have now, I can remember since I was six years old. It was not that I made them. A profession, a trade, a necessary occupation, something to fill and employ all my faculties, I have always felt essential to me, I have always longed for, consciously or not. During a middle part of my life, college education, acquirement, I longed for, but that was temporary. The first thought I can remember, and the last, was nursing work."—Florence Nightingale (Cook, 1913a, p. 106)

In Nightingale's time, nurse leaders were graduates of the Nightingale School who were frequently hand-picked and mentored by Florence Nightingale herself. One of these Nightingale nurses was Florence Lees. When the Crown Princess of Prussia met with Nightingale in the Franco-German War of 1870–1871 with a request for a nurse leader to take charge of nursing at a German war hospital, Lees was Nightingale's choice and her visits and reports from German hospitals highlighted the inadequacy of these facilities. Her feedback and Nightingale's advocacy resulted in the establishment of training schools for nurses in Germany that advanced the quality of care there (Cook, 1913b, pp. 203–204).

Lee's career continued in 1878 with her appointment to "organize District Nursing in London" (Cook, 1913b, pp. 253–254). She held the post for several years and efficiently ensured that sick poor populations received the same level of care as their wealthier counterparts (Cook, 1913b). Lees followed in the footsteps of another Nightingale nurse, Agnes Jones, who was named Lady Superintendent of the Liverpool Infirmary in 1865. Jones and 12 Nightingale nurses under her supervision began reform of workhouse nursing. The Liverpool Infirmary housed 1,200 men in its filthy wards. There was little attention to cleanliness with residents wearing dirty shirts for several weeks and bed linens unchanged for months. The diet was inadequate. Jones developed political savvy in dealing with these issues and gaining the support of the doctors and administrators. Her work was so successful that her nurses were also asked to provide care on the women's wards too. In less than three years, Agnes Jones brought order to the Liverpool workhouse and her success was emulated by Lees and other Nightingale nurses who expanded the influence of nursing in numerous facilities throughout the world (Cook, 1913b).

Today, 400,000 registered nurses are employed in formal and informal leadership roles in the United States and are the largest group of healthcare leaders in the workforce. They have opportunities to influence the individual patient experience, improve population health, enhance quality/cost effective care, and promote team vitality/joy in work. In 2017, 16 national nurse leaders met for two days to discuss how nurse leaders can develop and maintain work environments that meet the measures of IHI's Quadruple Aim. The group decided to use a theoretical framework developed by Dr. Jeffrey Adams as the foundation for their work. This framework is called MILE ONE—the Model of the Interrelationship of Leadership, Environments and Outcomes for Nurse Executives (Batcheller, Zimmerman, Pappas, & Adams, 2017).

MILE ONE includes three concept areas: nurse executives influence professional practice and the work environment; positive work environments and professional practice influence organizational and patient outcomes; and organizational and patient outcomes influence nurse executives. Discussion centered on nursing leaders' role in promoting research about the practice environment, advocacy for patient-centered care, serving as change agents in crises, and acquiring resources for care to underserved populations. Four major priorities were delineated:

1. Nurse leaders must develop "interprofessional models of care that optimize the use of resources, scope of practice, and determinants of health" (Batcheller, Zimmerman, Pappas, & Adams, 2017, p. 205).

2. Nurse leaders must create efficient and effective systems by basing standards of practice on evidence and evaluating outcomes based on national benchmarks. Past effectiveness is not always indicative of future success (Batcheller, Zimmerman, Pappas, & Adams, 2017, p. 205).

3. Nurse leaders must realize that clinical nurses may change positions more often today, and in the future and they must support a shared vision and professional practice model that will encompass the interprofessional team and collaborative team-based care (Batcheller, Zimmerman, Pappas, & Adams, 2017, p. 205).

4. Nurse leaders must "fully partner in national policymaking and improve the health of the population" served and "create a health system that brings joy to both patients and clinicians" (Batcheller, Zimmerman, Pappas, & Adams, 2017, p. 206).

Many nurse leaders have focused on cost reduction, quality improvement, and promoting patient-centered care. Now, their skill set must expand to include team vitality and joy in work. Millennial nurses don't just want to master their current roles and are focused on planning for future career opportunities. Effective nurse leaders will help this generation of nurses to develop a career plan and coach them to achieve their future goals. The nurse leader who realizes the importance of coaching will develop more engaged nurses who are involved in professional development activities that benefit their patients, the organization, and themselves (Sherman, 2017, p. 154).

Opportunities for nurse leaders continue to expand and evolve beyond facility walls and into the community, the region, the nation, and the world. The future of healthcare is unsettled, and these nurses are integral to achieving the goals of the Quadruple Aim. Each is unique, and their massive success reflects Nightingale's commitment to improving the experience of care for individuals, improving population health, reducing healthcare costs, and promoting team vitality and well-being. Their stories will be interspersed throughout this book to illustrate how their professional journeys positively impact the future of nursing and healthcare, including the Quadruple Aim. Let's meet them now.

Introductions—Why Did You Become a Nurse?

- Lya has been a nurse for 10 years and is a leader in a healthcare organization, where she is responsible for multiple roles, including nursing research, professional development, transition to practice, and Magnet designation. Lya's story illustrates the lasting impact of nursing on families in crisis.

  "I became a nurse because of my personal experience with our son. I was thriving in the music world and was a university professor as well as accompanist and church musician. I became pregnant and we had our son, Ian. My husband and I agreed that I would stay home with our son and teach piano students in the evening when I could have his help. When our son was seven weeks old, he stopped breathing on me while I was changing his diaper. We ended up in the pediatrician's office and then ultimately in the ED with him. After a long night, Ian was diagnosed with Tetralogy of Fallot with Pulmonary Atresia. He lived for 21 months and passed away during his third open heart procedure. During all of our hospital stays, I always demanded to be involved in Ian's care and daily rounds at the bedside. It was because of our persistence that the Pediatric ICU (PICU) started rounds with patients' families at the bedside. After Ian passed away, I kept feeling a 'nudge' to at least explore nursing as a career. So I did—I took prerequisites and then completed a fast-track BSN program. I knew that I wanted to work in the PICU. I made an agreement with myself that I would stop pursuing this nudge if I was coming home crying each day. I tailored all of my electives and classwork around pediatrics and even completed a rural rotation with pediatric cardiologists around our state. I got a job in the PICU and loved every minute of it. As a nurse, and now an advanced practice nurse, I really feel that I can not only empathize with the caregivers, I certainly *know* how they feel and what they need. Sometimes, patients and/or families just need a few extra minutes to share their story. In those brief minutes a nurse can really connect to patients and/or families and foster that relationship that helps guide the care for them. Ian's purpose in life was not only to give us joy, but to teach us unconditional love. I honor him every day by accepting patients for who they are, meeting them where they are, and being their best advocate.

"After a few years, I went back to school and finished my MSN and DNP. In addition to my nursing administration role, I practice as a pediatric nurse practitioner and love the time I get to spend caring for children and their families. I still spend a lot of time outside of work in the music community by accompanying and directing music at our church. This helps keep me focused and grounded!"

- Sheri has been a nurse for 15 years and began her career in acute care. She is currently in a senior leadership role for a professional organization nationally and is proud of receiving her DNP. Sheri became a nurse "to impact others and see how I could make a difference in a person's life at the most vulnerable times."
- Aislynn has been a nurse for 16 years and is a leader in a healthcare organization where she directs ambulatory care and is responsible for "nursing scope of practice across 65 diverse ambulatory practice sites." As a DNP, Aislynn also functions "as adjunct faculty for four colleges/universities in BSN, MSN, and

DNP courses." She was attracted to nursing at a young age: "As a young child I knew I wanted to be a nurse. I always wanted to help people and felt led to nursing. I originally thought I might like to be a nurse anesthetist but after entering nursing school believed I wanted more patient interaction. I started as a nurse on an Acute Medicine inpatient unit and have never looked back."

- Kati has been a nurse for eight years in neuroscience critical care and cardiac medical-surgical units. She currently has an MSN degree and a busy schedule. Kati works as a PRN in cardiac medical-surgical and is active as a leader in education/ professional development in independent practice and as a nurse entrepreneur. Nursing was a logical choice for her: "I went into it for very practical reasons: I enjoyed education, the medical field, and wanted something with a reliable job outlook/security and consistent paycheck."

- Jann's nursing career has spanned 43 years, beginning in pediatrics and culminating in her current role as a leader in an academic education organization and national professional organization. Jann uses her PhD and nursing knowledge to promote continuing medical education and interprofessional continuing education and collaboration. Her reason for pursuing a nursing career is "I love caring for patients and families. I have always been focused on how to help people get better and/or get the highest quality of life regardless of their health conditions. I love to be a positive part of the healthcare team and serve as the point of contact for coordination/management of care."

- Kari has been a nurse for 38 years, attaining a BSN and MS degrees and certification in a nursing specialty. She currently is a leader in education as a nurse entrepreneur and co-editor of a professional nursing journal. Her reason for seeking a career as a nurse is succinct and meaningful: "To help others use the best of science and caring."

- Cathy is celebrating 40 years in nursing and uses her BSN, master's in health administration (MHA), and certification as a leader in a healthcare organization to supervise professional development programs. She also serves as liaison to local schools of nursing. Her reason for choosing nursing reflects her passion for the profession: "As a child I loved the idea of helping others recover from injuries or illnesses; I saw nurses caring for patients and wanted to be them. As I grew up, I realized it was more than just the technical skills I loved but the critical thinking involved and challenges that influenced my decision to become a nurse. I recognized the flexibility of nursing, there is something for everyone, no matter your passion. I feel it is important for nurses to realize too that over time and professional growth their passions may change."

- Lienne has been a nurse for 47 years and after employment in parent-newborn nursing became a leader in academic education. After a distinguished career and academic progression from BSN to MSN to PhD, Lienne teaches part-time periodically. She became a nurse because she "wanted to work with mothers and babies; eventually to be a nurse-midwife."
- Andrea became a nurse 41 years ago. She is a family nurse practitioner who now serves as a leading policy advisor for a national professional organization. A healthcare advocate with a PhD in nursing, Andrea says her reason for becoming a nurse was based on practical experience about the profession: "My mother was a nurse; my first job was a nurse's aide."
- Brenda has been a nurse for 37 years and is currently an independent consultant who focuses "on strategic transformation in healthcare, academics and bio tech." A proponent of continuing education, Brenda began her career with an associate degree in nursing and ultimately attained a PhD in nursing. Her story reflects her love for her mother: "My mom worked nights as a nursing assistant in an extended care home, she worked really hard for minimum wage. She was an awesome person and I thought I could carry on for her and nursing seemed a good career. I started as a two-year RN, worked full-time my entire career while going to school to get my BSN, MSN, MBA and PhD in nursing."
- Joseph began his nursing career 15 years ago. He is certified with an MSN degree and currently is a leader in a national professional nursing organization. Joseph's career path began in high school. Here is his story: "In high school, I had to volunteer at a hospital and found it very enjoyable. In my senior year of high school, my sister had a complicated pregnancy, and I stayed with her in the hospital to keep her company. Watching all the 'cool' things the nurses were doing was amazing. One day in the cafeteria I saw a male nurse. I never knew men could be nurses. I was sure that was what I wanted to do. My niece was born at one pound, three ounces, and watching the medical staff work together to ensure a safe patient outcome was invigorating. I knew I would not want

to work in OB, but I started to explore the other options I could pursue."

- Debra began her nursing career 30 years ago as an associate degree nurse. Since then, she has earned a BSN and a master's in liberal arts (MLA) degree. She has served in professional development education roles and is currently a leader in a healthcare organization, specializing in accreditation and regulatory readiness. She became a nurse because her "grandmother worked as a scrub tech in the OR while I was growing up and I always wanted to help other people just like her. When I was 14, I had a ruptured appendix and ended up in the hospital for a lengthy stay. I was impressed and inspired by the nurses that cared for me on a day-to-day basis and I knew then that was my calling."

- Courtney has been a nurse for 11 years, beginning as an associate degree graduate and progressing to a PhD in nursing. She is currently a leader in a state behavioral health organization in the dual roles of adult psychiatric mental health nurse practitioner and family nurse practitioner. Courtney became a nurse based on family advice: "My grandmother was my inspiration for becoming a nurse. I was unsure of my path after graduating high school and my grandmother suggested I become a nurse. It has been the best and most rewarding decision I have ever made."

- Jean has practiced nursing for 42 years and specializes in nursing professional development. Her education journey began as a diploma graduate and progressed to a PhD in education. She currently is a leader in a national healthcare organization that partners with healthcare facilities/groups by providing a competency-based system that achieves positive patient outcomes. Jean's reason to become a nurse is concise: "to care for others."

- Sue has been a nurse for 44 years. She currently is a PhD–prepared professional development specialist in a regional healthcare organization and her leadership extends to research studies and mentoring graduate students. Sue's reason for entering the nursing profession is remarkable: "I don't have a very traditional entry into nursing. I didn't have any role models in the family. All my family, immediate and cousins, are all in business or computers. I grew up with three other siblings—all boys—so I played with the boys and somehow when they got hurt, which we all did, I'm the one that took care of them, including stitching up a younger brother's leg with regular needle and thread at about age 10. The doctor said I did a great job when he saw it later and said he wouldn't redo it since I had done such a good job. We also didn't run to the doctor for everything. If you got hurt you took care of it yourself, if you could. Doctors cost money. We were told we will go to college and have a career, so when it came time to go to college and I was filling out the forms for what to study, my mother suggested nursing, so I checked the box. It has been a fabulous career for me. Flexible for babies and their lives and varied for my interests."

- Pam celebrates her 50th anniversary as a nurse in 2019! She is a leader in professional development for a professional organization and a continuing education expert at the national level. Pam has a PhD and is a sought-after speaker nationally. She became a nurse based on her "long standing desire to work in a healthcare environment; combining my skills in leadership, communication, strategic planning and thinking, and working with others (I never had a vision of being a front-line provider, but always wanted to be involved at the leadership, decision-making level)."

- Mary is an MSN–prepared certified nurse who has been in the profession for 30 years. She currently is a professional development leader in a healthcare organization. Mary's story about why she became a nurse is intriguing: "I've always been interested in health, promoting healthy lifestyles, and helping others be the best they can be. I wanted a career that would allow me lots of flexibility and the opportunity to continually learn new things, challenge myself, and grow professionally. I also liked the fact that nursing offers the opportunity to balance work and home life without a complete setback in your career. When I was young and starry-eyed, I really wanted to be a flight attendant and travel the world. Somebody told me that some airlines looked for flight attendants who were also nurses. I thought this was another great reason to pursue nursing!"

- Michael has been a nurse for eight years. He has an MSN degree and has dual certifications in psychiatric-mental health nursing and professional development. He is a leader in professional development in a healthcare psychiatric organization. His journey into nursing has been long and rewarding: "I began my journey as a giver of care in 1979 while working in a community group home for adults with developmental disabilities. Most of these persons had been recently discharged from a lifetime of living in the state hospital system. As a young person, this experience helped to establish my personal paradigm which has attracted me to the vulnerable, at risk, and persons in need. Out of that mindset, there evolved a sense of social justice which has emerged as a passion for advocacy in some form or another. Over the course of my life, I have generally filled the role of caregiver as a CNA, but at some point, I felt the drive to level up to become a registered nurse. My wife has been a nurse as long as I've known her, and she has certainly been my inspiration for excellence in nursing. There was the draw of better pay and the hope that I would be more relevant in society because the professional RN is unchallenged as the most respected of all professions. I can't help but think that my hesitation to become an RN until I was 50 years old was related to a deep fear that I was not smart enough or that I did not have the ability to make critical decisions. Worse yet, I had a lingering dread that I lacked the ability to truly care."

- Dawna has been a nurse for 23 years. She has attained a PhD in nursing education and has specialized in "nursing education in both academic and practice arenas." Currently, Dawna is a leader in international nursing consultation and a nurse entrepreneur. Her reason for selecting a nursing career illustrates how a personal health crisis can result in positive future outcomes: "At age 22, I was a young military wife. My husband and I had two daughters born with congenital heart defects. My first daughter died after 72 hours of hypoplastic left heart. My second daughter had open heart surgery at six months of age for Tetralogy of Fallot. At a very young age, I learned how the lack of healthcare knowledge for medical terminology and navigating the healthcare system could render individuals helpless, confused and overwhelmed. My husband was often deployed, and I was left to make critical decisions with little or no understanding of what was being communicated by the healthcare team. When I turned 25, my daughter, now three years old, became stable enough for me to begin my journey toward the nursing profession. I was compelled to gain fundamental knowledge to better understand and act upon the healthcare challenges our family faced or may face in the future. Once I entered the profession I learned, and continue to learn, how moral and ethical principles of humanity drive our profession. The 'why' I became a nurse has evolved. Over the years, I have reflected on 'why' I continue to be a nurse. I continue to be a nurse because I believe I can make a difference in the patient population we serve. The 'patient' looks different with each role or responsibility we hold, be it an individual family member, a patient care assignment as a bedside nurse, or future patients as we teach and mentor emerging nurses at local, national, and international levels."

- Loressa's nursing career has spanned 40 years. She has a PhD in nursing, holds two professional certifications and currently serves in an executive leadership position in a national/international nursing organization. Loressa's decision to become a nurse reflects the influence of nurses on patients and families: "I was exposed to nursing at age 16 when my mother became gravely ill and experienced frequent hospitalizations. I was so impressed with the nurses who seemed smart, confident, and passionate about helping my mother *and* her family. Despite being on track to pursue a degree in engineering, I made a career choice my senior year of high school and applied to nursing school. A decision I have never regretted."

- Susan has been a nurse for 34 years, beginning with a BSN and progressing to a PhD in nursing. She also has two certifications and currently is a leader in an academic education organization and a professional development specialist at a healthcare organization. Her nursing journey reflects the influence of family on career choice: "My mother and grandmother were nurses, and I always admired their knowledge, competence, and compassion. I wanted to contribute in a meaningful way, and also wanted to ensure my independence and ability to be flexible and self-sufficient."

- Becky began her nursing career 36 years ago. She is certified in professional development and has two master's degrees— MSN and MHA. Becky currently is a leader in professional development for a large healthcare organization. Her choice to be a nurse reflects her love for her mother: "I observed my mother caring for family members throughout my life. Although she was not a nurse, she took numerous loved ones into our home and demonstrated daily compassionate, loving and respectful care for their physical, emotional and spiritual needs. Empathy and compassion were demonstrated on a daily basis in our home which raised my awareness of the needs of others everywhere. My mother never discussed the satisfaction caring for others brought her, but it was easily observed in her actions."

- Niki has been a nurse for 20 years. She began her education

with an associate degree in nursing and has attained a BSN
and master's degree along with two certifications—in her
neuroscience specialty and professional development. Niki is
a leader in education in a healthcare system and she became
a nurse for a positive purpose: "If you ask, most people have
an aspiration for their lives. They strive to make their family
proud or to serve our country. I want to make a difference in
people's lives. I want to positively impact those around me. Their
interactions with me also influence me to become a better version
of myself."

- Judy's 40-year career in nursing began in an associate degree
  program and culminated with a PhD in nursing. She is a leader
  in nursing education in a large healthcare organization and is
  certified in her specialty. Judy selected nursing as a career after
  much deliberation: "To help others while they are sick. My
  mother was a nurse, so I took a long time deciding if nursing
  was really what I wanted or was I just following my mother's
  footsteps. I decided that I really wanted to become a nurse."

- Kathy began her clinical practice 30 years ago in neuro/neuro-
  trauma. She has a PhD in nursing and currently is a senior leader
  in a national/international nursing organization. Her decision
  to seek a nursing career was a thoughtful one: "Desire to be
  in clinical practice/health professions; wanted better work/life
  balance than physician role (at the time I was in school)."

- Cathleen has been a nurse for 36 years practicing in pediatrics
  and professional development. She has two certifications and a
  PhD in nursing. Cathleen is a leader in professional development
  in a pediatric healthcare organization. Her reason for becoming
  a nurse was based on seeing her relatives' healthcare choices:
  "Many nurses and doctors in the family."

- Jacqueline has an MSN and two certifications. She specializes
  in nursing leadership with clinical experience that encompasses
  medical/surgical, critical care, and emergency nursing. She is
  currently a nursing director in a large regional healthcare system
  with responsibility for general medical nursing units and an
  observation unit, including the medical intensive care unit. She
  also supervises dialysis, IV team, diabetes education, and the
  eICU teams that support inpatient units. When she became a
  nurse 36 years ago, Jacqueline took her mother's advice: "My
  mother suggested I try being a nursing assistant when I was in
  high school. Back then you didn't need to be a certified nursing

assistant, the long-term care facility would teach you through classes and on-the-job training to be a nursing assistant. I applied for a job as a nursing assistant and was immediately accepted. I absolutely loved it, I enjoyed helping older people who needed our care. They were kind and appreciative, and I loved getting to know them. If they were not cognitively capable of participating in their care, I knew I was still doing something important, something not many people were willing to do, and I was making a difference in their life. When it came time to choose a career, I never really considered anything other than being a nurse. After 36 years, I would do it all over again."

- Tina has been a nurse for 30 years. She holds dual certifications and has an MSN. Tina has specialized in nursing professional development and pediatrics and is a leader in professional nursing organizations. Her reason for becoming a nurse 30 years ago began in her childhood: "As a child my favorite book was *Florence Nightingale,* so I always was interested in being a nurse. The allure of being a nurse stayed with me and I wanted to help people and make a difference in lives and the community."

- Charlene became a nurse 42 years ago as a diploma graduate. Subsequently, she progressed educationally to a BSN, MSN, MS in education, and a doctorate in nursing (DNS). Charlene holds two certifications and is currently a full-time tenured professor. Her first love was teaching and nursing became a logical choice as a career: "Growing up I always wanted to be a teacher, I even had my own 'school' set up on the porch at our home. When working with the guidance counselor in my high school, I expressed my desire to become a teacher. However, in the early '70s teaching positions were limited. I was then advised to become a secretary or nurse. I loved the sciences and people so I thought nursing was a good fit. Although nursing was not on my radar at 17 years old, I have not regretted one minute of that life-changing decision. How was I to know at the time how important teaching is to our patients, families, and our profession?"

- Mike has been a nurse for 20 years, beginning with an associate degree and advancing to an MSN. He is currently the chief operating officer for a heart institute in a large Midwest health system. His reason for seeking a nursing career reflects his support for others: "To help others who are most vulnerable and need our help. It has been an honor to help people survive and continue their lives, but also been just as much an honor to

be with families and help them with support when their loved
ones don't make it. Not too many jobs on this planet put you in
contact with caring for others and the impact we can have in our
profession and the well-being of fellow human beings."
- Maureen has been a nurse for over 25 years and will complete
  her doctorate in nursing (DNS) in 2019. She has specialized
  in administration and is currently a leader in a national and
  international nursing credentialing program. Her reason for
  selecting a nursing career mirrors that of Florence Nightingale:
  "I always wanted to be a nurse. I spent my summers with my
  grandparents, my grandmother had COPD. I used to help her
  with her bath and nebulizer treatments. They always called me
  their little nurse; I never considered being anything else."

Nightingale's Philosophy and Today's Nurse Leaders

Florence Nightingale was a woman of faith and her faith permeated all
aspects of her life. She expressed her philosophy in her own words: "God's
scheme for us was not that He should give us what we asked for, but that
mankind should obtain it for mankind" (Cook, 1913a, p. 479). Nightingale's
philosophy of nursing was expressed by her biographer in *The Life of Florence Nightingale* in this way: "Miss Nightingale was the founder of modern
nursing because she made the public opinion perceive, and act upon the
perception, that nursing was an art, and must be raised to the status of a
trained profession" (Cook, 1913a, p. 445).

How do today's nurse leaders feel about the nursing profession and
what is their nursing philosophy? This is best expressed in their own words.

- "The patient is the center of our care."—Lya
- "Education is the key to a successful nurse. You must continue to
  grow, evolve, and seek out opportunities to learn."—Sheri
- "Nursing is caring, truly caring, for people. No matter what
  position I have been in my career from bedside nurse to clinical
  head nurse, to educator, to director of nursing, the core of what I
  do is always caring for people."—Aislynn
- "Nurses are humans too and require just as much intentional care
  as the patients in our keep."—Kati
- "Nurses have a unique perspective that blends and leverages the
  needs and perspectives of patients/families/communities with the

expertise and performance of clinicians, teams and organizations. Nurses are the water in the stream of healthcare: we move and adapt to our surroundings and the skills of our colleagues, teams, and system to advocate and care for our patients/families."—Jann

- "It is an honor and a privilege to be a nurse to help others, often during their most challenging times."—Kari
- "Nursing is both an art and a science; it is a process which embodies the heart, soul, mind, and imagination."—Cathy
- "It is a blessing to be a nurse and be able to help others … and in my career that was with expectant/new parents and their babies, and then with nursing students. What a privilege to share a birth experience."—Lienne
- "Nurses leading change to advance health."—Andrea
- "'Beginnings are scary; endings are usually sad, but it's the middle that counts most'—Steven Rogers"—Joseph
- "Nurses are awesome, they are the answer to fixing our health system. They are natural process engineers and the bedside nurses have the solutions to our problems. The job of leaders is to make sure the structures and processes are in place to allow the nurses to achieve the outcomes. In a nutshell … *servant* leadership."—Brenda
- "At this time in my career its to guide RN colleagues in their professional development."—Jean
- "My philosophy is to inspire others and provide useful, nonjudgmental information to everyone regardless of their position."—Debra
- "Making a difference in people's lives, helping them reach their goals. Like when a patient wants to go home to die, we forget it's their life, it's their body, they get to decide. Or a patient doesn't want lifesaving intervention, we forget, it's their choice and we have to support and assist them to get that choice. We are the facilitators and advocates."—Sue
- "I believe that nursing has a unique position in the healthcare system to impact delivery of quality healthcare and improving health outcomes for individuals, families, and communities. (Note that I did not use the word 'patient'; I really believe in the bigger vision for nursing!)"—Pam
- "Nursing looks at the whole patient and the big picture and pulls together the whole team to provide the best care to the patient."—Mary
- "Commit to continued professional growth through ongoing

education and certification; and to base nursing practice on evidence and the highest of professional standards."—Courtney

- "Establishing and sustaining dynamic and integrated human experiences that result in a feeling of genuine meaningfulness and relevance in whatever way that consciously and unconsciously makes sense to the person."—Michael
- "Nursing is a calling to serve humanity."—Dawna
- "Nurses are at the center of the healthcare team and in this position uniquely understand the holistic approach needed to address individual patient *and* public health needs."—Loressa
- "I believe the nurses are the center of the healthcare system. Nursing is a profession central to yet unique from all others in its body of knowledge, application of theory, and influence on outcomes. It is nursing's responsibility to advocate for its ongoing role and recognition."—Susan
- "The nursing profession provides me an opportunity to incorporate my core values of love, Christian compassion and healing principles into my daily life." Becky
- "We are here to guide and enable those that seek a higher state of well-being through the continuum that is modern healthcare."—Niki
- "Nursing is not just a job but a calling that requires advanced knowledge and skills from numerous disciplines to provide care to those in need."—Judy
- "I believe fundamentally nursing is a relationship with a person and his/her family (in the broadest sense) with the ability to promote health, prevent illness, manage or cope with disease, and die well without prejudice or bias throughout all levels of society."—Kathy
- "Embrace every opportunity as a nurse, when you have the privilege of helping/witnessing/sharing vulnerable moments in people's lives when you make all the difference in their experience."—Cathleen
- "As a nursing leader, put the patient at the center of every decision you make. I'm not sure if that is a 'real' philosophy or more of a guiding principle, but when I do this, I make the best decisions. Very simple. Closely aligned with that, as we make decisions about patient care, I always think—is that how I or a loved one would want to be treated?"—Jacqueline
- "Nursing is the opportunity to make an impact, provide change and be an advocate for whoever is in your sphere of influence."—Tina

- "Nursing is caring and competence, but it also entails nursing leadership at any decision-making table where a nurse's voice should be heard, be it the bedside to the boardroom."—Charlene
- "Caring for others as I would want my family to be cared for."—Mike
- "Nursing is humbling. I am honored and grateful to be able to do the work. If I can help one person that day, then, it was a good day."—Maureen

How Does This Fit with the Quadruple Aim?

This diverse group of today's nurse leaders are men and women of different generations who are employed in multiple positions in different locations and organizations. Their backgrounds and paths to nursing are all different, but they each impact the success of at least one of the four aims in their practice as Florence Nightingale and past nurse leaders improved the experience of care for individuals through education, improved the health of populations, reduced healthcare costs, and improved provider work life (team vitality). The issues are complex, and these nurse leaders are at the vanguard of current and future change within the healthcare environment.

4

Quadruple Aim Goal 1

Improving the Experience
of Care for Individuals

"In watching disease, both in private houses and in public hospitals, the thing which strikes the experienced observer most forcibly is this, that the symptoms or the sufferings generally considered to be inevitable and incident to the disease are very often not symptoms of the disease at all, but of something quite different—of the want of fresh air, or of light, or of warmth, or of quiet, or of cleanliness, or of punctuality and care in the administration of diet, of each, or of all of these. And this quite as much in private as in hospital nursing."—Florence Nightingale (Nightingale, 1992, p. 5)

Florence Nightingale was a visionary who realized that individuals' health required more than solely focusing on inpatient and disease treatment. She advocated for prevention and sanitation by caring for well individuals in the community and ensuring that their home environments were also healthy with pure air, pure water, efficient drainage, cleanliness, and light (Nightingale, 1992, p. 14). In addition, Nightingale also advocated for attention to diet and careful observation of patients to ensure that they experienced safe care. She also stressed the importance of courtesy when communicating with patients: "Always sit down when a sick person is talking business to you, show no signs of hurry, give complete attention and full consideration" (Nightingale, 1992, p. 28). Such advice today would benefit how individuals experience their care.

Although this chapter focuses on improving the experience of care for individuals, it is important to remember that each Aim is interdependent, not independent and all must be considered together because each impacts the others (Butterworth & Sharp, 2016). Some progress has occurred since 2008, but more remains to be done in the future.

Improving the experience of care for individuals has focused on satisfaction with care for hospitalized patients. The Centers for Medicare and Medicaid Services (CMS) requires hospitals caring for Medicare patients to report patient satisfaction data via the HCAHPS (Hospital Consumer Assessment of Healthcare Provider and Systems) system. This data on patient perspectives is analyzed by CMS and publicly reported on the Hospital Compare website where individuals can review critical aspects of the hospital experience to make informed choices about their quality of care (Centers for Medicare and Medicaid Services, 2018).

Armed with this information, individuals must be engaged in their healthcare and empowered to take charge of their own health, including adherence to the plan of care, healthy lifestyle changes, and preventive health screenings (Butterworth & Sharp, 2016). Even with patient-centered medical homes and availability of low-cost or free clinics in the community, this does not always occur. How can individuals be mobilized to participate fully in their own health?

A promising approach is interprofessional education and collaboration of the healthcare team with the patient at the center of the team. Health care and patient education has often been conducted in silos where interdisciplinary teams interact with each other and the individual but focus on their own responsibilities and performance—not on the performance of the entire team and inclusion of the patient and family/significant others. This parallel approach does not always produce positive results for the individual. For the individual to truly benefit from interactions with the healthcare team, the team must be interprofessional and contain everyone who has knowledge that can impact the individual's health and care. This may include support staff—patient care assistants, housekeeping staff, dietary personnel, and others who have information applicable to the individual's health. Disciplines, such as medicine, nursing, physical therapy, respiratory therapy, etc., must teach and learn from each other and keep the individual at the center of the team. Individuals are also no longer passive recipients of care. They want active involvement and to be heard as they share concerns and needs. This model encourages these individuals to gain control of their health and learning needs and creates an interprofessional learning environment where there are no silos, only a true collaboration by everyone for the individual's benefit (Chappell, 2016).

The role of the nurse is vital in improving the individual experience of care. As members of the most trusted profession, nurses are in a unique position to influence how individuals perceive their healthcare experiences (National Nurses United, 2018). The Institute of Medicine realized in 2010 that reformation of the United States healthcare system would require transformation of the nursing profession to respond to individuals' concerns and needs via patient-centered care. Nurses are involved in all aspects of healthcare "from health promotion, to disease prevention, to coordination of care, to cure—when possible—and to palliative care when cure is not possible" (Institute of Medicine [IOM], 2011, p. 4). Nurses must transform their practice to ensure the right care at the right time to individuals with health needs and the Institute of Medicine recommended changes to better align nursing practice with the needs and perceptions of individual patients/clients. These recommendations included the following.

1. Nurses should practice to the full extent of their license and education by removing scope-of-practice barriers for advanced practice nurses (IOM, 2011, p. 9).

2. Nurses should have opportunities to lead and disseminate collaborative improvement activities (IOM, 2011, p. 11).

3. Nurses should have the opportunity to complete transition-to-practice residency programs upon graduation or when moving to new areas of clinical practice (IOM, 2011, p. 11).

4. Nurses should attain a baccalaureate degree to enhance their practice with a goal of 80 percent by 2020 (IOM, 2011, p. 12).

5. Nurses should attain doctorates to serve in faculty and research roles with the goal of doubling the number of doctoral-prepared nurses by 2020 (IOM, 2017, p. 13).

6. Nurses must be lifelong learners to competently care for diverse individuals and populations (IOM, 2011, p. 13).

7. Nurses must be prepared to lead change at all levels to advance health (IOM, 2011, p. 14).

8. An infrastructure to collect and analyze data about interprofessional healthcare workforce requirements must be developed (IOM, 2011, p. 14).

These recommendations were reviewed in 2015 when the Robert Wood Johnson Foundation requested the IOM (now the National Academy of Medicine) to address the progress of these eight recommendations and identify areas of emphasis for the Future of Nursing: Campaign for Action and its State Action Coalitions to pursue in the future (National Academies of Sciences, Engineering, and Medicine, 2016, pp. 3–4). Here are their results.

1. Removal of scope-of-practice barriers—13 states met criteria for full practice authority in 2011. By 2015, eight additional states granted full practice authority to nurse practitioners, 17 other states had reduced practice authority, and 12 others restricted practice. Although

progress was made in the five years after the original publication, more work remained to fully meet this recommendation nationwide (National Academies of Sciences, Engineering, and Medicine, 2016, p. 41).

2. Nurses leading and disseminating collaborative improvement activities—Interprofessional education and collaboration continues to expand with team-based care. By 2015, 75 percent of the State Action Coalitions included non-nurses as stakeholders because true interprofessional collaboration requires the work of all healthcare professionals. Measurement of this recommendation was "limited to counting interprofessional courses offered at the top 10 nursing schools" (National Academies of Sciences, Engineering, and Medicine, 2016, p. 145). The Campaign noted that this measure was not sufficient and that nursing leadership in collaborative improvement activities will require data about nurses' participation in courses and programs "in leadership, entrepreneurship, and management" (National Academies of Sciences, Engineering, and Medicine, 2016, p. 149).

3. Implementation of nurse residency programs—These programs have increased in health facilities and vary in length and content with many focusing on acute care practice and retention rather than on their impact on patient outcomes. The Campaign did not include a measure that tracks residencies in healthcare settings and recommended use of accredited residency models and greater focus on implications for patient outcomes from residencies (National Academies of Sciences, Engineering, and Medicine, 2016, p. 84).

4. Eighty percent BSN–prepared nurses by 2020—This will be a difficult recommendation to achieve by the target date. Employers prefer BSN–prepared nurses, but there are still large numbers of nurses prepared at the associate degree level. Community colleges and four-year universities are collaborating more to provide access to BSN education for graduates with associate degrees (National Academies of Sciences, Engineering, and Medicine, 2016, p. 74).

5. Double the number of nurses with doctorates by 2020—Lack of faculty continues to be a barrier to fully achieving this recommendation. DNP programs have increased faster than PhD programs from 2010 to 2015. Practice settings and roles of these nurses must be clarified to demonstrate their leadership "in clinical care, research, education, and other areas (including public policy and business)" (National Academies of Sciences, Engineering, and Medicine, 2016, p. 92).

6. Nurses' engagement in lifelong learning—Although interprofessional continuing education is promoted, no comprehensive data

exists about requirements for lifelong learning by nurses from states and health facilities. Competencies are variable, and skills are dependent on the environment and setting where nurses practice. The Campaign could not evaluate progress toward this recommendation but offered to coordinate discussion between nurses and other healthcare professionals to address opportunities for collaboration in addressing this recommendation (National Academies of Sciences, Engineering, and Medicine, 2016, p. 98).

7. Nurses leading change to advance health—The Campaign has focused extensively on placing nurses on health-related non-profit or corporate boards where they will have the opportunity to advance health in leadership roles. Although there has been an increase in nurses on boards, there has been less success in promoting nurses as leaders in key healthcare leadership positions. Data is incomplete about the influence of nurses as leaders in organizations as well as on boards (National Academies of Sciences, Engineering, and Medicine, 2016, p. 161).

8. Improving infrastructure for workforce data collection—Data has been collected within the health professions and the Minimum Data Set for nursing supply, demand, and education data is helpful in developing a workforce database. However, expanding data sources and sharing data are areas that the Campaign must promote to ensure comprehensive workforce data collection and analysis (National Academies of Sciences, Engineering, and Medicine, 2016, p. 172).

This interim review also resulted in additional recommendations beyond the original eight. These recommendations included the following.

1. Diversity in the workplace must be a priority. A diverse workforce reflects the population it serves, "including economic, racial/ethnic, geographic, and gender diversity" (National Academies of Sciences, Engineering, and Medicine, 2016, p. 11).

2. Nurses must have increased opportunities for leadership development and interprofessional collaboration. By expanding its alliances, the Coalition can promote leadership development programs that are interdisciplinary and help nurses play a valuable role in "interprofessional collaboration in care and delivery" (National Academies of Sciences, Engineering, and Medicine, 2016, p. 12).

3. Nurses must be involved in redesigning care delivery and payment systems. The Campaign should encourage nurses in employed leadership and executive positions to fulfill this recommendation in health systems, for-profit health clinics and insurance companies,

not-for-profit organizations like the National Quality Forum, professional groups like the National Academy of Medicine, and local, state, and federal governmental agencies that are health-related. Expansion of "metrics to measure the progress of nurses in these areas" is also essential (National Academies of Sciences, Engineering, and Medicine, 2016, p. 13).

4. The Campaign should gain support for its activities by communicating with "a broader, more diverse stakeholder audience" about progress toward the recommendations (National Academies of Sciences, Engineering, and Medicine, 2016, p. 13).

These recommendations are applicable to the IHI Quadruple Aim's objectives and should be considered as a component in their success.

Input from Today's Nurse Leaders

Florence Nightingale and early nurse leaders focused their efforts to improve the experience of care for individuals through the education of nurses who provided direct patient care. Today's nurse leaders also realize the importance of competent nurses in helping individuals navigate their own healthcare and wellness. They realize that the IOM recommendations are relevant for nurses to provide the best quality care for individuals and promote practice to the full extent of education and license; higher levels of education for nurses; residency and transition to practice programs; lifelong learning, including continuing education and certification; emphasis on diversity and inclusion; interprofessional education and collaboration; and developing nurses' leadership skills (National Academies of Sciences, Engineering, and Medicine, 2016).

Here is their perception and how they are addressing these IOM recommendations and improving the experience of care for individuals.

- "I was recruited for my current position in nursing administration. I like the role as it allows me to see and lead organizational projects that result in change—which ultimately affects patient care. To see a new nurse understand the 'why' for the first time is rewarding. To see policy change and practice change to affect patient care for the better is rewarding. I enjoy large projects and have been asked to lead our clinical ladder restructuring for our entire system. This gives me great pride that our CNO group has the trust in me to accomplish this enormous task, but it gives me the most pride in that we will be able to retain the best of the best nurses which will, in turn, allow us to give the best patient care possible."—Lya

- "I am humbled to see so many programs wanting to validate their nurse residency and APRN fellowship programs."—Sheri
- "My current role is an executive position and comes with many challenges around change management and people management. Over the past two years I have led restructuring of departments, formalized nursing leadership forums so that middle managers have support and resources and created multiple forums where front line staff have access to Senior Leadership to share concerns or challenges. In addition, we have really increased the ambulatory focus on the social needs of our patients. This work is transforming how we care for patients."—Aislynn
- "A nurse from Australia messaged me and said that because of my podcast, she picked up on signs her terminal patient was deteriorating and was able to call the family in time for them to say one last goodbye. When I get messages like that, they mean a lot to me."—Kati
- "Building new and innovative approaches to continuing education and performance improvement that enhance the work of clinicians and teams. I want to positively impact the care that individuals and teams provide to patients/families and communities—and how to make systems work to achieve these expectations."—Jann
- "Seeing others grow and accomplish more than they thought possible. Seeing their expertise and confidence grow—for patients, families and nurses."—Kari
- "I frequently speak to high school students about career options and after speaking to them, they express awe at what nurses actually do compared to what they see on TV. When I receive a thank you from someone; whether it comes from a patient, family, nurse, or student it reminds me that I am making a difference."—Cathy
- "I enjoy teaching and interacting with nursing students; being able to teach a course one to two times a year is fun and keeps my brain active (keep learning!)."—Lienne
- "I enjoy so many aspects of my role as an educator. I do sometimes miss patient care, but I have found joy in helping other nurses enjoy their lifelong learning."—Joseph
- "The ability to connect with the nurses who actually provide

direct care and be a role model and mentor for them and to enable structures and processes for the bedside nurses to provide the very best care for patients. I profoundly believe in the evidence that supports the Magnet program and do everything in my power to embed them in organizations I work with. My direct contact with the bedside nurses and new grads is important to me and I transfer my personal and professional power to them, so they can make positive outcomes happen!"—Brenda

- "Mentoring others. As I near the end of a wonderful nursing career I get great satisfaction out of meeting new nurses and working with colleagues to create opportunities to learn and grow in their profession."—Jean
- "I love to educate and guide at all levels in the healthcare field. I have a passion for working with our new nurses in particular to ensure that they get a foot up as they begin their professional journey. If I can inspire one person, my mission has been accomplished."—Debra
- "Making a difference—either in an individual's life—staff or patient or on a bigger scale—in nurses' lives and doing meaningful work."—Sue
- "Inspiring others to be creative and innovative in providing professional development opportunities to strengthen teams, teamwork, and positive outcomes for patients and healthcare teams."—Pam
- "I really get a lot of satisfaction out of the consultative role that NPD (nursing professional development) practitioners serve in. When a colleague comes to me and says, 'We've noticed this problem and we need help figuring it out,' I become really energized! I love trying to break down an issue, get to the root of what the problem is, and work to put into play possible solutions."—Mary
- "Knowing that I am able to make a difference in my patient care and lives."—Courtney
- "There are several events that give me pride, but the most powerful is when a patient thanks me and is glad I was their caregiver. There was once a man about my age who had been in the psychiatric unit for a couple of weeks to support his recovery from a severe crisis related to schizophrenia. As he was being discharged, he stopped at the exit and walked briskly over to me. I was not sure of his intent because his gaze was intense, and his countenance was like that of someone on a mission. With an

intense gaze, he reached out his hand and said, 'Michael, thank you for not treating me like a schizophrenic.' What more can one ask out of life than to feel like you've made a difference in the life of someone who is a social outcast and has lived a lifetime with little hope of experiencing a full and satisfactory life!"—Michael

- "Currently, I work at an international level. I am most satisfied when I have shared current and relevant best practices with my international colleagues to improve patient care outcomes."—Dawna
- "Every day I report to work for an organization whose sole purpose is to elevate the image and work environments of nurses in the U.S., and even the world."—Loressa
- "I would say the freedom to be creative, and the opportunity to help others reach their potential or at least move to their next phase of their professional development. I love to break down complex ideas and then build them back up in a way that makes sense and helps others understand and apply new ideas. I enjoy informal consulting and working with faculty as they face challenges in the classroom, clinical, or online learning environment."—Susan
- "Whether it is a patient, family member, student, young or older nurse—I experience immense satisfaction from helping others through something they find difficult. Currently—my role brings me into contact with people in positions of high influence and power within our organization. Working in a healthcare system as large and diverse as ours presents many organizational challenges which I may not always understand. However, my courage arises from the fact that I am paid to be an expert in education. It is an expectation that I will always speak the truth about educational issues, regardless of the outcome."—Becky
- "When I was a newly practicing nurse, the healthcare culture was still of strict servitude to physicians and you either performed nursing tasks well or 'got ate.' I respect the ability to contribute to the knowledge and skill base of new nurses. I want them to flourish in the new interprofessional team approach to nursing. Bedside nursing takes moxy in the face of long hours, physical tasks, and higher demands. I feel I have made an impact when nurses not only want to stay in their current field of nursing but start expressing the desire to become certified or ask about volunteer activities. I strive to fill their brains with knowledge

and their hearts with compassion and spirit for their own bedside practice."—Niki

- "In my current role I really enjoy helping bedside nurses and other clinical nurse educators to learn and grow in our profession. I enjoy learning and sharing information that can help my co-workers to perform more efficiently with greater knowledge and skills to provide better patient outcomes."—Judy
- "Ability to positively impact the professional practice of nursing globally; mentoring others/nursing leaders; developing new programs to meet evolving needs of registered nurses; interprofessional collaboration with medicine and pharmacy."—Kathy
- "Knowing that I make a difference in the lives of others."—Cathleen
- "I love it when I can improve the processes of care. When I can make things easier for nurses and improve patient outcomes at the same time. I am also very proud of our culture of servant leadership, caring for each other, and humbly serving the patient. We can set aside politics, egos, and competition and achieve a cohesive team working towards a common purpose, having a great place to work and take excellent care of our patients."—Jacqueline
- "I enjoy developing others and providing the tools for others to grow and advance themselves."—Tina
- "My intrinsic reward is working with our future nurses in my faculty role and paying my profession forward. Seeing my students succeed and make a difference in the lives they touch—how can one's life get any better! By sharing my knowledge, experiences, and passion, I hope to incite students to give compassionate, safe, quality care to every patient they encounter and to have a voice as an advocate for the patient/family unit and the profession of nursing."—Charlene
- "Overseeing the development of programs that optimize care for our patients and seeing my colleagues act upon those developments to provide the best care to the hundreds of patients who trust their care to us on a daily basis in the heart institute."—Mike
- "Being able to promote the profession of nursing. Helping nurses understand the vital role they play in improving patient outcomes, to think of nursing as a profession (not a job) and to move beyond 'I am just a nurse' and saying 'I am a nurse'"—Maureen

These powerful insights demonstrate that Nightingale's spirit is still alive in current practice by nurse leaders to improve the experience of care for individuals and advance nursing practice. There is more work to be done, but the foundation is strong.

5

Quadruple Aim Goal 2
Improving the Health of Populations

"The very elements of what constitutes good nursing are
as little understood for the well as for the sick. The same
laws of health or of nursing, for they are in reality the
same, obtain among the well as among the sick."—Florence Nightingale (Nightingale, 1992, p. 6)

Florence Nightingale devoted much of her life to improving the health
of populations, beginning in the Crimea where she focused on improving
the life of British soldiers. While caring for the soldiers' physical needs,
she determined that their social and psychological needs were equally important, but usually neglected. British soldiers were frequently drunk and
demoralized. Their officers displayed indifference to the conduct of their
troops. Nightingale believed that soldiers' behavior would improve with the
correct approach and she set out to prove it. Her strategy was to create a
reading room for recovering troops and promote education for the soldiers.
She also educated any officers who would listen "to treat the soldiers as
Christian men" (Cook, 1913a, p. 277). Her example encouraged the English
people, including the Royal family, to send books, games, newspapers, and
artwork that were shared with soldiers via a reading room and a schoolroom
at Scutari. Her sister, Lady Verney, handled the collection and delivery of
these and other items at Nightingale's direction. Lady Verney described this
process in a letter to a friend: "I don't know whether Mrs. Milnes told you
how hard we worked to send off boxes for F.'s education of the army! Let me
tell you, Ma'am, to instruct 50,000 men is no joke. Finally, I thought a little
art would be advisable, and had a number of prints stretched and varnished
which are to be my subscription towards the improvement of the British
army!" (Cook, 1913a, pp. 280–281).

Florence Nightingale's initial idea grew and evolved over time. The
Army supported reading and recreation rooms that improved soldiers' lives.

Her success is summed up by her biographer that "no modern barrack is deemed complete without its regimental institute, with recreation room reading-room, coffee-room, and lecture-room, while means of out-door recreation and shops for various trades are also provided" (Cook, 1913a, p. 397). Nightingale's original idea has improved the lives—physical, social, and psychological—of countless British soldiers and is an excellent example of improving the health of an at-risk population.

Current Populations

Selection of a population should be paired with creating a better care experience for that population's members and reducing healthcare costs. Two common types of populations are enrolled populations and regional/community populations. Enrolled populations are usually "a group of individuals who are receiving care within a health system or whose care is financed through a specific health insurance plan or entity" (Whittington, Nolan, Lewis, & Torres, 2015, p. 267). These individuals may be health system employees, health insurance plan members, patients within a specific practice, or participants in an accountable care organization (ACO). These population members can be calculated based on their enrollment. Regional/community populations are delineated geographically. These populations contain sectors defined "by common needs or issues, such as low-birth-weight babies or older adults with complex needs" (Whittington, Nolan, Lewis, & Torres, 2015, pp. 267–268). There is no common source of care for these individuals and some may lack insurance and receive no care at all. For these reasons, it is difficult to count this population and adequately address its health needs.

Another approach with regional/community populations would be monitoring its subset over time. Individuals with congestive heart failure in a state or county could be tracked to determine their health status as well as care experiences and per capita costs of providing care. Primary care innovations, such as patient-centered medical homes, community clinics, retail health providers (e.g., pharmacies), and telehealth where care is not tied to a certain location enable these population members to obtain consultation and care that they would otherwise not receive and use (Berwick, Nolan & Whittington, 2008).

Health care organizations and providers must collaborate with other stakeholders (e.g., business leaders, policy makers, community agencies, public health departments, public officials, school leaders, local employers, etc.) to enable at-risk populations to gain knowledge about how to improve their health and the opportunity to take actions that will enable them to lead a better, healthier life. Stakeholders will vary based on the population needs and benefits. These stakeholders include: "(1) those who would benefit if the health, healthcare, and per capita costs improved for the population; (2) those who could directly or indirectly influence the necessary changes; (3) those who would champion the spread of successful changes; and (4) those who had access to the data and measures that would drive Triple Aim results" (Whittington, Nolan, Lewis, & Torres, 2015, p. 270).

Managing an At-Risk Population

Diabetes is a chronic, costly disease that affects approximately 150 million individuals in the world currently. Complications include blindness and visual impairment (diabetic retinopathy); kidney failure; heart disease; diabetic neuropathy; and foot disease that may lead to amputation. Diabetes treatment includes dietary control, exercise, and medication—oral agents or insulin. Preventing its onset and managing its progress are feasible with weight reduction and walking 30 minutes daily (World Health Organization, 2018).

Beginning in 2014, a longitudinal study on diabetes care management began in Louisiana, a state with the greatest death rate from diabetes in the United States. Patient-centered medical homes (PCMH) previously discussed have the potential to meet Triple Aim measures, including improvement of health for at-risk populations. Although medical students have had opportunities to learn about PCMH and care management, other professions must be incorporated into interprofessional teams in practice settings. The study used two urban settings—a "hospital-based ambulatory clinic for internal medicine residents and an urban faculty practice that consisted of faculty in the disciplines of family medicine and internal medicine" (Coleman, McLean, Williams, & Hasan, 2017, p. 29).

44 students were assigned to each of these two sites with a minimum of four disciplines at each site. Students included medical students (#15); physician assistant students (#3); nursing students (#8); social work students (#2); pharmacy students (#8); and internal medicine residents (#4). Team members stayed at their sites for up to two academic semesters and each received training in their own discipline first followed by interprofessional education. The population consisted of 36 adults from ages 18–70 with uncontrolled Type 2 diabetes. Each student had assigned roles that weren't exclusive and could be performed by students from other disciplines as needed. The interprofessional team and the individual client

jointly developed the plan of care (Coleman, McLean, Williams, & Hassan, 2017).

All team members were housed in the same location and teamwork extended to coaching individual clients to take actions toward a healthy lifestyle. Although 40 adults with uncontrolled diabetes agreed to participate, four did not complete any of the program. Students' teamwork skills improved significantly and the clients rated the program highly on communication, helpfulness and friendliness, ease of receiving care, and quality of care received. As an educational program, the Diabetes Medical Education Program could not pay for lab tests for clients. Many of this population was underserved and couldn't afford blood work or transportation for appointments. There was reliance on self-reporting of lifestyle changes and telephone conversations rather than face-to-face interviewing (Coleman, McLean, Williams, & Hasan, 2017).

This study of longitudinal care management illustrated issues impacting ambulatory care of at-risk populations. Recruiting clients was time-consuming and limited financial resources reduced clinic visits and laboratory testing. Clients who did not speak English were partnered with students fluent in their languages. Adherence to prescribed medications was also an issue for those who could not afford their medications and for those who neglected to comply with required doses. The majority of clients did make some healthy behavior changes because students encouraged group visits to exchange ideas, provided education on medications, and encouraged frequent contact with the participants. This program has added school-based clinics for teens with obesity and pre-diabetes. This study showed that interprofessional learning and collaboration within the PCMH model can benefit populations with chronic disease resulting in positive outcomes for participants and providers (Coleman, McLean, Williams, & Hasan, 2017).

As this study illustrates, some progress is being made in population health, although this progress must continue to impact the lives of populations in need.

Input from Today's Nurse Leaders

Nightingale and early nurse leaders employed a variety of approaches to support the healthcare needs of populations they served. Each population had different needs and required unique tactics and methods. They realized that success would be tempered by failure and that opportunities would be shadowed by challenges. Yet, they pressed on to achieve the goal of improved health for diverse populations.

Today's nurse leaders are also confronted by numerous challenges and opportunities as they support nurse colleagues to achieve success of the Quadruple Aim. Here are their perceptions:

- "The biggest challenge for me is that our organization is growing exponentially, and senior leadership wants everything done as soon as possible. With process change, there are many players that need to be involved (process, practice, policy, education) and it always feels like we are pushing new projects out way too fast and too many at a time. I think this is the way of healthcare and we have a challenge to find a way to streamline the process to assist the bedside staff."—Lya
- "I never thought I was smart enough to get a doctorate. I was always 'just' a nurse. I know now that I am more than 'just' anything and I can create change."—Sheri
- "There are two main challenges in this role. First is keeping all the balls in the air. About a year ago, I was sitting in on an interview for another executive level nursing position. The candidate asked what some advice would be for a new nurse executive. One of my colleagues said, 'learn to juggle.' This is very true. I often have days full of meetings and each one is a completely different topic from the next. It takes a lot of organization and focus to keep it all going. The second challenge is keeping perspective. Change is hard and although my teams have made wonderful change, it can be easy to lose that perspective every now and then. Stepping back and looking at all we accomplished is a wonderful thing to do. Certainly, there is a lot ahead of us, but remembering what we have done thus far is important!"—Aislynn
- "There's a lot I'd like to do, but not enough time or resources to do so independently."—Kati
- "Many healthcare systems, institutions and organizations assume that continuing education is optional, and not an essential element in providing and promoting quality care, clinician and team self-worth and employee/staff retention. My most significant professional achievement is longitudinal. I am the nurse 'at the table' in discussions about continuing medical education (CME), continuing education in the health professions, accreditation and board certification discussions."—Jann
- "Time—mostly others' lack of time to focus on their own development."—Kari
- "The most significant challenge in my role is that of being a

change agent; it is also my biggest opportunity: encouraging collaboration for bedside competencies and inter-disciplinary education and yes inter-disciplinary competency. Most professionals want this opportunity but don't know how to go about it, they are afraid to change from the status quo."—Cathy

- "Opportunity: to be able to continue teaching without the hassles of fulltime work is most rewarding."—Lienne
- Opportunity: "Being part of a network that is modernizing nursing laws and regulations—federal and state." Challenge: "Elected officials who lack knowledge and/or empathy for vulnerable persons."—Andrea
- "I commit to large complex projects that are often 'against all odds' endeavors. I enter the healthcare organization in a role to assess, plan and fix things and see the project thru to completion then exit. I have a unique style, knowledge base, experience, education and professional portfolio that wraps up into a skill set that is coveted in our healthcare industry. I choose who I work with, the locus of control is definitely with me. I always have tried to improve systems and processes that needed to be fixed even before I knew it was called performance improvement. I always get excited by challenges that make most people run from the building screaming."—Brenda
- "Challenge: Planning for retirement which includes succession planning. There needs to be some education and work aids out there that help an RN transition out of nursing (just like there are aids to transition from academia TO professional practice). Opportunity: Share experiences and wisdom. Listen to other generations of nurses and their perception(s) of practice no matter where they are. Work on projects that support, develop and enhance the profession."—Jean
- "As I am new to my role, understanding and correlating the State and Federal regulations and making them understandable for our front-line staff as well as leaders. Being able to link our practice to the required elements is essential."—Debra
- " The challenges, as in, not good use of my time and skills are the routine tasks in the job that I wish I could have a secretary do, that require no skill from me but can be very time consuming, as in signing people up for routine classes for onboarding, so my time could be better spent on something more meaningful. Management often jumps to solve every employee behavior with education. The good thing about being a more experienced

educator is, I will ask to do an assessment of the situation first and if it's NOT a lack of knowledge/skill I remind the manager it's not an educational issue, but an accountability issue—their problem, not mine. Education should be based on assessment of need—employee self-assessment, system wide issues, manager assessment of staff, coworker assessment of the team, and educator assessment, so that bringing all these views together should lead to a pretty accurate picture of what the needs are, what priority do the needs have and what plans can be made for resolution of those needs. This has been a big change in the organization, getting the organization to be proactive not just reactive. We have done a system wide assessment each year now which helps. The last issue is weak follow through. We are so eager as an organization to throw together an intervention that we don't finish the whole cycle of following up to see, did our plan get our desired outcome? So, I'm always bringing outcomes up and trying to train the folks I can influence to think of measuring the outcomes."—Sue
- "The 'we've always done it that way' mentality or 'urban myths' that get in the way of current, evidence-based standards."—Pam
- "Getting others to realize the power of nursing professional development (NPD), and what our true role is. So many times, other leaders come to me (or my team) and say, 'We want you to do this…' without really identifying if that is the best solution to the problem at hand. I would rather them engage us in a collaborative way and analyze the issue and potential solutions together."—Mary
- "Finding time to volunteer for community events due to my work schedule. I sometimes work 14-hour days and I'm not always available to assist with community events. I feel that community involvement is critical to preventative healthcare. It also allows practitioners an avenue to give back, an opportunity to see first-hand how their work impacts the community, and an opportunity to network."—Courtney
- "As I find my niche as a professional nurse, opportunities have been emerging that allow me to take advantage of my strengths leading me to be more relevant in my role as a nursing professional development practitioner, within the organization as an advocate of mental health, and within the community and state as an advocate for suicide awareness and prevention."—Michael
- "My most significant challenge is time management. My passion,

commitment, and interest in improving frontline care delivery often leads me to accept assignments, opportunities, or projects without consideration of the resources needed for completion. There is much to do, and I am a visionary and futuristic person. I tend to look at 'what can be' without consideration of 'how we get there'!"—Dawna

- "The political climate and focus on America's healthcare needs are misaligned. Accessible healthcare is a right of every American and nurses are in a unique position to advocate and represent those needs."—Loressa
- "As I suspect many others may say, having time to give each project or challenge the attention it deserves is an ongoing challenge. There is also a widening gap between current teaching practices and expectations of Gen Y and Gen Z learners in the academy and the workplace. The need for faculty development is urgent. I also worry about retaining young qualified nurses at the bedside beyond one year of practice."—Susan
- "Budget constraints have reduced the educational staff to the point where we are unable to integrate the knowledge into the complex environments of clinical practice."—Becky
- "We are change agents. I struggle with having enough time to devote to every task I want to complete. I would like to have more of an impact on those in our community."—Niki
- "My greatest challenge in my current position is to educate and convince senior leadership of the value of continuing nursing education. Educators are valued when something goes wrong, but as an educator I struggle to show the daily value of the education provided to the nurses and how this contributes to the patient outcomes."—Judy
- "Most significant challenge: resource demands for credentialing programs to meet growth strategies; speed/flexibility/innovation to market. Most significant opportunity: ability to influence the profession of nursing for the future, including international impact."—Kathy
- "Resource allocation for continually updating nursing practice in a dynamic healthcare arena."—Cathleen
- "I think it is how to effectively use technology without creating more work for nurses. We can't let technology drive our practice, it has to inform and support our practice. It seems in the era of electronic health records, social media, and the digital world in general, it is easy to lose touch (literally) with the patient."—Jacqueline

- "The challenge is I become so enthusiastic at times I overextend myself; I want to be involved in too many projects. The opportunity is I love my job and the opportunity to think outside the box and develop programs."—Tina
- "My worry is the growing need to graduate increasing numbers of new nurses. Unfortunately, there are many constraints seen nationally that are barriers to admitting the numbers of students we need in the future to serve the public's healthcare needs. Preparing the nursing workforce of the future is limited by clinical site availability for student clinical placement, significant faculty and nurse retirements, educational costs, and the complex needs of patient requiring more nurses now and into the future."—Charlene
- "This would be the depth and breadth of my areas of accountability and responsibility. I often tell the story that as a bedside RN I cared for two patients and their families 12 hours a day for three days a week. In my current role, I oversee the delivery of care on a grander scale and with that comes a coordinated effort with everyone paddling in the same direction. I find pride in observing team members delivering care, sharing results of a test, scheduling a procedure, interacting with patients and families."—Mike
- "As with any nursing leader job, there are always multiple competing priorities. My first commitment is to advocate/support for my staff, so they are able to do their jobs—certainly both a challenge and an opportunity."—Maureen

It is evident that today's nurse leaders confront both challenges and opportunities as they are on the frontline of healthcare changes that impact population health. Some are involved in interpreting and improving legal and regulatory issues that impact underserved populations. Others address complex projects and improve systems that change care delivery in multiple environments. Others play an essential role in preparing practitioners and facilitating lifelong learning. They believe, as Nightingale did, in evidence-based practice that results in optimal outcomes for members of diverse populations.

6

Quadruple Aim Goal 3
Reducing Per Capita Costs of Healthcare

> "This place [1 Upper Harley Street] is exactly like the administering of the Poor Law. We have cases of purely lazy fits and cases deserted by their families. And my Committee have not the courage to discharge a single case. *They* say the Medical Men must do it. The Medical Men say *they* won't, although the cases, they say, *must* be discharged. And I always have to do it, as the stop-gap on all occasions."—Florence Nightingale (Cook, 1913a, p. 136)

Nightingale wrote this to her father about her first position as a nurse leader in London and it is eerily reminiscent of today's managed care system. When the author first began clinical practice, a fee-for-service payment basis was in place that reimbursed the quantity of care provided. Physicians were encouraged to order multiple tests and hospital stays were longer because there was no incentive for the hospital or physician to dismiss patients no longer requiring hospitalization. Under that system, children were hospitalized for seven days after a routine appendectomy and mothers and babies stayed in the hospital for 72 hours after normal delivery. Today, either would be laughable. Nightingale's approach to discharging patients staying beyond their need for care fits well with current healthcare practices. Managed care has been around since the 1980s with the objectives of providing quality healthcare and outcomes by managing utilization and costs for enrolled populations (Medicaid, 2018).

Government Reimbursement

Government involvement in healthcare reimbursement related to quality care has increased since the inception of managed care organizations.

74

Today the Centers for Medicare and Medicaid Services (CMS) has implemented a Value-Based Purchasing Program (VBP) that pays participating hospitals for inpatient services based on the quality of care provided and withholds or reduces payments based on outcome measures. These measures include patient safety, patient experience, mortality and complications, healthcare-associated infections, efficiency and cost reduction, and process. This program has expanded to skilled nursing facilities and in-home health agencies in nine states representing different geographic areas to reimburse based on performance of quality and more efficient care delivery. A Value Modifier is expanding in 2018 to include, in addition to physicians, nurse practitioners, clinical nurse specialists, and certified registered nurse anesthetists "who are solo practitioners or in groups of 2 or more eligible practitioners" who are reimbursed via Medicare payments for performance on cost and quality measures. CMS also uses its Hospital Readmissions Reduction Program (HRRP) to reduce payments to participating hospitals with excess readmissions within 30 days for Acute Myocardial Infarction (AMI), Chronic Obstructive Pulmonary Disease (COPD), heart failure, Coronary Artery Bypass Surgery (CABG), pneumonia, and elective total knee or total hip arthroplasty (CMS.gov, 2018).

HCAHPS (Hospital Consumer Assessment of Healthcare Provider and Systems) was mentioned in a previous chapter and also serves a purpose beyond supporting consumer choice through public reporting. Since 2007 hospitals receiving payment from the Inpatient Prospective Payment System (IPPS) have been required to "collect, submit and publicly report HCAHPS data in order to receive their full IPPS annual payment update (APU)" (Centers for Medicare and Medicaid Services, 2018). Failure to report HCAHPS results and other required quality measures results in reduced payment (APU). HCAHPS results also are used in the Patient Experience of Care domain in the Value-Based Purchasing Program and poor scores may adversely impact reimbursement for participating hospitals (Centers for Medicare and Medicaid Services, 2018).

These programs are designed to improve the experience of care for individuals, quality of care for individuals and populations, and per capita cost reduction of healthcare. Adjustments are made annually to achieve these outcomes. Progress has been made although more remains to be done.

Nurse Leaders and Financial Savvy

Nurses in leadership positions, particularly in professional development, are beginning to financially quantify their (and their staff members) contributions to the organization's bottom line and strategic plan initiatives. It is no longer enough to ensure employee education and competency. As healthcare facilities feel the impact of potential and actual reduced government reimbursement on their financial stability, all departments must validate their worth to the organization to maintain viability in the face of budget and staffing cuts. Lack of nurse leaders and professional development practitioners to support learning and practice needs of front-line nurses will adversely impact care delivery for individuals and patient populations and, in the long run, may result in higher per capita costs for turnover, orientation, and errors of omission or commission. Nurse leaders in these roles are beginning to use financial calculations, such as benefit-cost ratios and return on investment, to substantiate their contributions to quality patient care and cost avoidance that benefits their organization's fiscal stability (Opperman, Bowling, Harper, Liebig, & Johnson, 2016).

Population Management and Cost Reduction

Cost reduction cannot be achieved alone but should be combined with population management and a learning system that supports ongoing success. The population must benefit from reduced per capita cost, whether it consists of members of an organization enrolled in a health insurance plan or community members with common needs. Selecting high-risk populations with complex health needs can reduce overutilization of expensive emergency services for both these individuals and the healthcare organizations. In other communities, poor health makes it hard for local populations with chronic diseases to maintain an acceptable standard of living. Many of these individuals have difficulty accessing services because of lack of transportation and community-based clinics. Cost reduction is also important to these populations and their community stakeholders (Whittington, Nolan, Lewis, & Torres, 2015).

The health of employee populations and community populations requires investment by organizations and local coalitions that addresses the causes of poor health including socioeconomic factors. Oversight functions require "(1) those who would benefit if the health, healthcare and per capita costs improved for the population; (2) those who could directly or indirectly influence the necessary changes; (3) those who would champion the spread of successful changes; and (4) those who had access to the data and measures that would drive Triple Aim results" (Whittington, Nolan, Lewis, & Torres, 2015, p. 270).

Integration of services continues to be a significant issue and no organization or government agency has been able to assemble the resources and accept responsibility for achieving IHI's measures. The integrator's role will be pivotal in defining the purpose, coordinating with stakeholders, and promoting testing and learning to achieve Quadruple Aim measures. The integrator ensures that the purpose statement includes cost reduction, population health, and individual experience of care in the local area to involve stakeholders. Focusing on population subsets with similar needs will help stakeholders use interventions to address these needs. This is not an easy process due to populations with chronic illness exacerbated by substance misuse and/or mental health issues. Services and resources may not be readily available or integrated at the local level (Whittington, Nolan, Lewis, & Torres, 2015).

It is always best to begin with a small test using a pilot population before full-scale implementation of services and resources. Cost measurement could reflect the total cost of care per member of the population monthly or the utilization rate and/or cost of hospital services, including emergency department visits. Fulfilling the purpose requires a "portfolio of projects and investments to address the challenge" (Whittington, Nolan, Lewis, & Torres, 2015, p. 285). These projects may include health coaching, annual health risk appraisal, patient-centered medical home usage, redesigned services for at-risk complex populations, partnership between healthcare and community organizations, and improved access to care. Each project should have a designated leader to manage daily activities and a data specialist should be included to regularly check progress and determine if population level outcomes improve with local project outcomes. Some organizations have had success in reducing cost per participant using the above approaches and establishing a framework for further testing. (Whittington, Nolan, Lewis, & Torres, 2015).

Government Influence on Cost Containment

The Centers for Medicare and Medicaid Services (CMS) play a significant role in hospital and provider reimbursement.

Hospital Value-Based Purchasing Program

In 2010, a provision of the Patient Protection and Affordable Care Act created the Hospital Value-Based Purchasing (VBS) program under the direction of CMS. This program continues today and focuses on improving quality and safety of care while enhancing the patients' experience of care. The 3,000 hospitals who participate in this program are encouraged to (1) reduce or eliminate adverse events that result in harm to patients; (2) use evidence-based protocols and standards to enhance patient outcomes; (3) transform hospital processes to improve the experience of care for patients; (4) increase transparency about care to consumers; and (5) receive recognition for providing cost-effective, high-quality care (CMS.gov, 2018).

The Hospital VBP program rewards hospitals for quality, rather than quantity, of patient care services. The program is funded by reducing Medicare payments for participating hospitals by a percentage allowed by law. In 2018 this percentage is 2 percent. This percentage is distributed to hospitals based on their performance as value-based incentive payments. Each participating hospital receives Total Performance Scores (TPS) based on outcome measurement, such as "mortality and complications, healthcare-associated infections, patient safety, patient experience, process, efficiency and cost reduction" (CMS.gov, 2018). Each hospital is scored twice on each of these measures—once for achievement and once for improvement. The hospital's final score is the higher of these two scores. The Total Performance Score for each measure reflects hospital performance compared to all hospitals and improved performance compared to performance in a prior baseline period (CMS.gov, 2018).

Quality outcome measures change to reflect importance to patients and providers. In FY2018, care transition was added to ensure that patients understood their care when discharged. Quality domains and weights were "Clinical Care (25 percent), Patient and Caregiver Centered Experience of Care/Care Coordination (25 percent); Safety (25 percent), Efficiency and Cost Reduction (25 percent)" (CMS.gov, 2018).

Hospitals that do not demonstrate achievement or improvement in selected care measures will be penalized by funding reduction. The VBP program has been extended to physicians and other eligible professionals based on performance in designated quality and cost measures by rewarding those who provide quality care at a lower cost. The Home Health Value-Based Purchasing (HHVBP) model began in 2016 in all Medicare-certified home health agencies in nine states representing each geographic area of the United States. This Model rewards quality of care and efficiency and tests whether greater incentives for improved quality will lead to better outcomes. The Skilled Nursing Facility Value-Based Purchasing Program (SNF-VBP) begins in FY2019 and uses incentives based on reducing hospital readmissions within 30 days of discharge from the skilled nursing facility. Payment incentives will be based on individual performance and comparison to other skilled nursing facilities in the United States. All skilled nursing facilities reimbursed under the SNF Prospective Payment System are eligible for performance incentives (CMS.gov, 2018).

Hospital-Acquired Conditions (HAC) Reduction Program

This program saves Medicare approximately $350 million annually by reducing payment to hospitals where more patients have hospital-acquired conditions. The HAC Reduction program was implemented as part of the Patient Protection and Affordable Care Act and in FY2015 hospitals in the lowest 25 percent of performance in reducing hospital-acquired conditions were penalized with a one percent payment reduction. Payments are adjusted when hospital claims are paid. Measures are based on the Centers for Disease Control and Prevention (CDC), the National Healthcare Safety Network (NHSN) and Healthcare-Associated Infections (HAI). These include "Central Line-Associated Bloodstream Infection (CLABSI); Catheter-Associated Urinary Tract Infection (CAUTI); Surgical Site Infection (SSI) (colon and hysterectomy); Methicillin-resistant Staphylococcus Aureus (MRSA) and Difficile Infection (CDI)" (CMS.gov, 2018).

Hospital Readmissions Reduction Program (HRRP)

The Hospital Readmission Reduction Program (HRRP) was established in 2012 under the Patient Protection and Affordable Care Act to improve healthcare for Americans by connecting the quality of care in hospitals to payment for services. Since hospital readmission rates differ across the country, this program provides an opportunity to improve care quality and save money for taxpayers while offering financial incentives to providers for reducing unplanned readmissions. This financial incentive promotes improved care coordination and communication while collaborating with patients and caregivers about post-discharge planning. The measures evaluated under HRRP are "Acute Myocardial Infarction (AMI); Chronic Obstructive Pulmonary Disease (COPD); Heart Failure (HF); Pneumonia; Coronary Artery Bypass Graft (CABG) Surgery; Elective Primary Total Hip Arthroplasty and/or Total Knee Arthroplasty (THA/TKA)" (CMS.gov, 2018).

The program measures hospital performance by establishing the excess readmission ratio (ERR) from the hospital's performance for each of these measures based on a ratio for expected/planned readmissions. The ERR for each measure determines the hospital's payment adjustment factor. This determines the payment reduction for ERRs above the median ERR in the hospital's peer group. The hospital's payment adjustment factor is subtracted from 1.0000 and multiplied by 100 to obtain a percentage. If the payment reduction is 0.97, the formula is 1.0000−0.97 = 0.03 × 100 = 3.0% payment reduction.

Unplanned readmissions within 30 days of discharge from the initial admission are counted whether the readmission occurred at the same facility or a different acute care hospital. Hospitals have a 30-day period where they can review and correct their ERR calculations for HRRP. They cannot send corrections to the claims data or add new claims to the data (CMS.gov, 2018).

Future Implications

Government involvement in healthcare reimbursement will continue. CMS considers these three programs an opportunity to assess quality, encourage transparency, and tie improvement to value-based payment in inpatient settings. Implementation in home health and skilled nursing facilities are a logical step in the future. Since involvement in all three programs can be complex, CMS is working to simplify requirements while providing financial incentives to improve the value and quality of care for individuals (CMS.gov, 2018). This is an ongoing journey requiring careful monitoring of care delivery and data that is comprehensive and user-friendly. A partnership between payers, including the CMS, healthcare organizations, providers, and the public must contribute to its success.

Regardless of what happens with the current healthcare environment, cost containment will continue to be significant in reducing per capita costs of care.

Input from Today's Nurse Leaders

Florence Nightingale and her fellow nurse leaders understood the importance of efficient, cost effective provision of care. Today's nurse leaders are confronted by multiple challenges in addressing cost issues that are unique to our times. It is important that all Aims be addressed interdependently, rather than separately, because each Aim affects the others. Let's hear from some of these leaders.

- "As the expectations for care become more closely linked to value-based care, the demand and need for independent, evidence-based continuing professional development that is competency-based and outcomes driven also increases. The need for quality continuing professional development professionals is going to be essential to supporting, clinicians, teams and institutions to meet those ever-increasing benchmarks."—Jann
- [most significant professional achievement] "Obtaining several million dollars of funding to support diverse students, financially and academically, so that they could be successful in a BSN nursing program."—Lienne
- "I also co-led with a physician partner a two-year electronic health record (EHR) system wide design and implementation and was successful in making sure nursing's voice was front and present to ensure positive outcomes for out-patients. I went to work for a large staffing corporation and designed a screaming innovation to increase revenue streams for this corporation with a focus on high quality as a counterbalance to their hunger for profits. I love collaboration and have forged lasting partnerships with academics to achieve Magnet."—Brenda
- "I think the workgroup around return on investment (ROI) has been my most significant achievement. The far-reaching impact that it has afforded us will impact generations to come. Additionally, it has strengthened me as an individual."—Debra
- "I went with a local group some months ago to testify before Congress as a caregiver of a person with Alzheimer's, on the lack of CMS resources to care for the person at home. There are lots of resources listed that are publicized as being available for caregivers of persons with Alzheimer's, but in fact the resources that are available have all kinds of stipulations that few people can meet. The CMS system really only pays for nursing home care. Even though everyone says, 'Oh yes, let's keep them at home, etc.,' few people really do it and few people can afford to do it unless they quit work. If you want to keep the person at home there is no funding, no respite, no resources and to institutionalize someone is very expensive compared to keeping them at home. So, we gave our testimony and that experience made me realize how much more influence I had and wasn't using. Because you quickly realize, funding drives development and funding goals determine what happens with a disease. In Alzheimer's we have spent billions on treatment. At present no treatment

cures Alzheimer's and a few drugs can slow it, but it eventually kills everyone or makes them so vulnerable that another health issue kills them. Almost nothing is being researched on causes, screening and prevention, even though it's listed as the biggest new trend in adult health. We are way behind on getting a handle on this disease. I had been following the funding allocations by the government regarding prevention and screening of a person at risk for Alzheimer's. I realized there is almost no funding in that area, so I found out when hearings were for the next round of NIH funding—biggest funder of Alzheimer's research—and went to testify again. But this time I brought 5 brain researchers, got a lobbyist and a handler and our little group testified in late March! I only knew one brain researcher and his specialty was not Alzheimer's. I contacted him, and he found the rest and, amazing to me, they all agreed to come to Washington and testify together on this issue. I'm learning a bit more about the process and navigating the testimony process. Anyone can testify, but if you want to make a difference, you have to testify to the committees that dole out the money at the right time in the funding cycle and you have to testify with the right Congressmen who can make a difference. That's where the lobbyist and handler come in. They know all this and guide you for a fee. You also need to learn who the organizational partners are—like in this case—AARP, so you can influence public opinion, the press, and move the public to your point of view to meet your goal which is the lobbyist's job. A lot more would have to be done to assure the NIH funding is changed to our view. Will our testimony change things? I hope so, since this issue is now getting in the news and on the radar. Of course, every time you do something big and audacious, you are changed forever, and it creates a platform for the next logical thing."—Sue

- "As a nursing professional development practitioner, one of the most frustrating challenges has been the lack of allotted resources and ultimate decision-making when it comes to developing educational activities. As organizations seek out ways to improve efficacy, those budgeted items that are not directly related to productivity are low hanging fruit for minimization. Education is not non-productive in that there is no obvious relationship to generating income. Hence the need for nursing professional development practitioners to vigilantly utilize return on investment (ROI) whenever possible. There seems to be less enthusiasm for seeking out the hidden connections between robust education and decreased waste and improved outcomes."—Michael

Today's nurse leaders acknowledge the financial challenges facing nursing and healthcare today in the United States. They also understand their responsibility to ensure safe, quality, efficient, and cost-effective care. Nightingale exemplified this throughout her life from facilitating cost-effective discharges at Harley Street to the development of the Nightingale School with funding from contributions of the British people for her service in the Crimean War. These funds were invested for her to create "an Institution for the training, sustenance, and protection of Nurses and Hospital attendants" (Cook, 1913a, p. 456). Her belief in the importance of nursing education and competency in patient care is reflected this statement from her biographer: "She had it in her mind from the first that her Training School should in its turn be the means of training elsewhere. She wanted to sow an acorn which might in course of time produce a forest" (Cook, 1913a, p. 461). Today's nurse leaders follow Nightingale's vision that lifelong learning for nurses positively impacts individual and population outcomes while reducing costs of care.

7

Quadruple Aim Goal 4

Improvement of Provider Work Life (Team Vitality)

[Conversations with Nightingale nurses] "But you are not looking well today. You have been sitting up too late? Yes? Then you must promise me to take better care of yourself." Or, "Are you careful to take regular meals? No? Then you must let an old nurse give you some good advice."—Florence Nightingale (Cook, 1913b, p. 308)

Work-related stress is not new, but it does adversely affect team functioning and resulting outcomes. Florence Nightingale's interactions with her nurses and students over many years reveal a maternal touch when addressing their needs. According to Derek Feeley, IHI President and CEO, "raising joy in work is a key strategy in the pursuit of the Triple Aim. Even in the best-performing healthcare organizations, staff burnout has a direct negative effect on the experience of care for the patient. There's also a correlation between high levels of staff engagement and high level of patient engagement. Staff are much more likely to be enthusiastic and positive about securing the best outcomes for patients when they feel supported, empowered, and respected" (Feeley, 2017).

Improvement in provider work life (team vitality) requires a variety of approaches and techniques beyond thanks for a job well done. Changes in care delivery models, such as interprofessional education and collaboration, enable the team to function in unity with the patient at the center, not compete with each other for resources (Chappell, 2016). Streamlining documentation enables team members to reduce the time spent charting rather than performing patient care. Standardized workflows can save time and provide higher quality care. Dedicating more personnel and financial resources allows the team to achieve positive outcomes for the individuals and populations they serve. Open team communication is essential to high-functioning teams and expanded nursing roles enhance the level of preventive care and coaching for chronic health conditions (Bodenheimer & Sinsky, 2014). A clinical learning environment enables members of different healthcare professions to learn from and teach each other for the benefit of the individuals they serve. This collaboration addresses everyone's learning needs and in turn supports positive patient outcomes (Chappell, 2016).

Each healthcare team member must develop methods to care for themselves, so they can care for others. In 1872 Florence Nightingale expressed her own approach to self-care through her faith by saying, "O my Creator, art thou leading every man of us to perfection? Thou knowest that throughout all these 20 horrible years I have been supported by the belief (I think I must believe it still or I am sure I could not work) that I was working with Thee who wert bringing everyone, even our poor nurses, to perfection" (Cook, 1913b, p. 243). How do today's nurse leaders care for themselves, so they can care for others?

- "I do mindfulness activities while at work. I get a massage regularly. I try to get at least six hours of sleep a night. I laugh— if you can't laugh at yourself or find something to laugh about, you're headed for disaster. I play music!"—Lya
- "Spend time with my family and friends. Exercise. Travel."—Sheri
- "Faith and family are very important to me. I work hard to maintain a healthy work/life balance. As a Director of Nursing, it is very easy to never stop working. Sure, I physically leave work, but I might bring home some things to review or open up emails on a Sunday afternoon to prepare for the week. I do these things, but I also am sure that I turn it all off and focus on what is important. Taking family vacations, even small trips camping, help me refresh. Getting my weekly dose of church is helpful as well. I use my drive to and from work to de-stress with music or devotionals. I also have a strong group of colleagues that support each other. We go out to dinner every few weeks. It is scheduled on our calendar and we can relax, enjoy some good food, and talk. Sometimes, we vent about the stress of the job or share our future goals. Either way, it is a great way to de-stress and support each other."—Aislynn
- "I see a counselor once a month. It helps me keep a healthy perspective, challenges me, and validates some of the complex emotions one walks through as they provide nursing care either directly or indirectly. I also am intentional about time away and focusing my efforts at work to things I am passionate about. I am

a huge proponent of practicing self-compassion, which enables me to provide authentic empathy without taking an emotional toll on myself. I think all of this together helps me prevent burnout and be mentally and emotionally present at work and at home."—Kati

- "I am still working on this—I actually find pleasure and fulfillment in other volunteer activities, in ballroom dancing, reading and doing puzzles. I also love to bake. I don't say 'no' often enough but believe that I am here to help others—so I take solace in knowing that my family, friends and colleagues can call when they need something."—Jann
- "I seek balance every day. I practice yoga daily and find joy in spending time with my dog. Looking into my dog's face I am reminded of the importance of being in the moment."—Kari
- "I firmly believe in leaving work at work. My computer goes off at 5 p.m. and I do not check my work emails until 0500 the next day. I am also involved in community activities that I find very relaxing: church, teaching English as a Second Language and of course there are my hobbies: boating (power boats and kayaking), fishing, target shooting, reading, card making—something for every season."—Cathy
- "Massage therapy at least once a month. Travel with my husband. Exercises to keep my shoulders and back more healthy."—Lienne
- "Keeping active—yoga, public transportation, water activities. Eating healthy—Weight Watchers."—Andrea
- "I try hard to have a work-life balance. I leave my stress and worries at the door. I laugh! I embrace my career and get involved in professional organizations to get excited about new opportunities."—Joseph
- "I am blessed to be married to the most wonderful human on earth who I call my archangel. I practice Reiki, yoga and Pilates on a daily basis. My animals, my beloved horse and Labrador, are a big part of me. Fundamentally, I believe that I must be strong, happy and healthy first, so I can help others and improve our health system. I have joy every day!"—Brenda
- "I plan outdoor time and exercise into every day. Sometimes it's just a walk or a bike ride."—Jean
- "I like to read, there is nothing better than curling up in a chair and letting your mind expand."—Debra
- "I do some self-care things really well—eat healthy, exercise, give myself Zen time. I'm not good at taking time off, but I'm working

on that goal. I tend to rob myself first to help someone else, especially with my time. For example, I'll come in on a day off to help someone, stay late at work if the unit is busy to help out for a bit, but I know in the process no one does my job for me."—Sue
- "Love to walk and read, so I take time daily to enjoy those refreshing experiences. I'm typically very even keeled, so stress management is not a problem. I do focus on healthy eating, rest, and time with friends. I'm also very comfortable in my own company and confident in my knowledge and skills."—Pam
- "I eat a healthy diet focused on fresh fruits & vegetables, healthy proteins, and high fiber. I run four to five days a week and do yoga twice weekly. I almost always get seven hours of sleep a night, attend church weekly, pray daily, and recognize God's awesome presence in my life! In my free time, I spend quality time with friends and family as much as I can and try to make the world a better place through volunteer service."—Mary
- "Eating healthy, exercising, reading, playing the piano, engaging in spiritual and meditation practices, and taking time to just have fun!"—Courtney
- "I rely on creating art in the form of songs. My band Sour Alley has produced three full-length albums with an international fan base that includes around 40 countries none of which prompts me to quit my day job. Creating is the tether that keeps me from the black hole of routine. If one is not careful, routine and the personal trauma that can come from seeing pain and death each and every day can become a pathologic emotional cancer. Sandra Bloom [2010; see References] wrote a wonderful exploration of art as a healing agent to the wounds we suffer as humans. Nurses are not immune and to keep soft and avoid becoming less soft, active self-care is required, not optional."—Michael
- "Admittedly, I have not mastered the art of self-care from a physiologic perspective. Most of my self-care is spent on intellectual growth and development. I enjoy reflection, journaling, and discovery of new and interesting concepts that help me mentor and support others to fulfill their dreams and aspirations."—Dawna
- "I carve out time every day to connect with myself thru meditation and physical activity. I recognize that I can only benefit others by caring for myself. That requires making time for my own professional development and growth, and most important, spending time with family and close friends."—Loressa

- "I have learned the hard way to take this seriously. I drink gallons of water and try to eat sensibly with lots of fresh food. I go outside every chance I get and enjoy walking, hiking, biking, yoga. I love to read and to cook for my family. I try, not always successfully, to sleep six to seven hours a night. I volunteer when possible and plan a vacation each year to somewhere I haven't been."—Susan
- "I am intentional about creating time for events, relationships and practices which bring me personal pleasure and satisfaction. Most of these are not nursing related! Flea marketing, an occasional massage or pedicure, a Saturday morning breakfast at the local diner with my husband, etc., all are things which give me something to look forward to. I also have milk and cookies every single night at 8:00 p.m.! (smiley face)"—Becky
- "You have to arm yourself with the strength to say 'no' and the knowledge to truly care for everyone. We are a global society; our little Midwestern town is blessed to have the diversity that we do right outside our front doors. We need to experiment with the healing arts of other cultures. We need to be able to take 'downtime' that is not considered to be a failure, but as a rejuvenation of our minds and spirits. When we embrace what is 'healing' to us, it spills over at the bedside as compassion for our patients and their loved ones."—Niki
- "Traditionally I have always put others first. With experience I have learned that if I do not care for myself, I will be unable to care for others. So, I now set aside time to exercise, to reflect, and to enjoy social occasions with friends and colleagues."—Judy
- "I exercise daily, eat well, strong family ties, take time to decompress/be alone when needed, spread work over several days on the weekend so I am not overwhelmed on Mondays."—Kathy
- "I 'fill up' by spending time with my own family."—Cathleen
- "First I make sleep a priority. With grown children that is easier now, but it makes everything else easier if you have sleep. Then, I prioritize exercise and activities I like to do, such as reading, knitting, etc. Finally, be sure to spend time with those you love. I know at the end of my life, I will never say, gee, I wish I would have spent more time at work!"—Jacqueline
- "I participate in activities that provide a challenge, for example, I run 5Ks, trail runs and mud races. I also volunteer for an animal rescue, an organization that gives back and it fills my bucket."—Tina

- "My mantra has always been 'family first.' Being with family allows me to re-center my priorities in life and appreciate where I have come from, where I am, and where I am going. With that, I like to focus on my gratitudes every day, it refuels the soul."—Charlene
- "Work/life balance. I don't take my work home with me—my computer stays at work. My family is my escape valve and their support enables me to do the work I do."—Mike
- "I practice mindfulness and remember to breathe!"—Maureen

Today's nurse leaders agree with Nightingale that it is important to care for yourself, so you can care for others. Her faith guided her and the results of her caring for others is illustrated by one of the Nightingale nurses who served in the Egyptian campaign of 1885. Sister Philippa Hicks met with Florence Nightingale for advice prior to embarking on her journey. She was treated to breakfast at Nightingale's residence and had another surprise when she boarded the ship. "Other nurses were going out in the same ship as I, and when we entered our cabins, we found a bouquet of flowers for each of us, attached to which was 'God-speed from Florence Nightingale'" (Cook, 1913b, p. 349). On her return, Sister Philippa was invited to stay at Nightingale's London home to complete her reports and then was welcomed at Claydon, Nightingale's country home where she rested for a month and visited with her mentor (Cook, 1913b). This is one example of many that illustrates Florence Nightingale caring for others and sharing her knowledge with them. The next chapter will explore how today's nurse leaders share their knowledge and advice with future nurses and nurse leaders as they pursue the Quadruple Aim.

8

Quadruple Aim
Nurses Leading the Way

"Let each Founder train as many in his or her spirit as he or she can. Then the pupils will in their term be Founders also."—Florence Nightingale (Cook, 1913b, p. 246)

Florence Nightingale coached and mentored her students and nurses to affect the individual experience of care, population health, and wise use of resources. She demonstrated motherly concern for both her students and practicing Nightingale nurses. Her advice was heeded and resulted in improvements in patient care delivery and the health of multiple populations.

Experience of Care for Individuals— Then and Now

The Liverpool Workhouse Infirmary in 1864 housed the poor of the city when they became sick. They were cared for by untrained nurses, many of whom were drunk, and most were indifferent to their patients' needs. Patients' clothes were dirty, and food was insufficient for their needs. When Nightingale was asked to intervene, she sent Agnes Jones as Lady Superintendent accompanied by 12 Nightingale nurses. Jones faced a formidable task but relied on Nightingale's advice and mentoring to succeed in reforming the Infirmary to the patients' benefit. According to Jones, "No one ever helps and encourages me as you do. I could never pull through without you" (Cook, 1913b, p. 128).

Today's nurse leaders are confronted by different challenges. Care coordination and care planning are vital to improving the quality of care for individuals in multiple healthcare settings. Care of individuals with complex health conditions requires coordination and collaboration of numerous practitioners and nurses are well suited to serve as care coordinators who involve the individual and his/her support network as active members of the care team. Individuals must understand the importance of behavioral change for health issues, such as diabetes and congestive heart disease. However, understanding is not enough. They must also be motivated and have the tools they need to change unhealthy behaviors. Nurses can help them find and use these tools by collaborating with other disciplines, such as nutritional services and exercise physiology. Care planning continues to be a challenge with a focus on standard care plans in electronic health records. Individualized care plans must be up to date and accessible to the entire healthcare team and the patient/client and his/her support persons. Everyone must be involved in modifying and updating the plan of care and everyone must adhere to its goals for it to be successful. Nurses are in a unique position to coordinate care and individualized care planning is an essential element as individuals make the transition between healthcare settings in hospitals and ambulatory care in the community (Ma, May, Knotts & Devito Dabbs, 2018). Today's nurse leaders can support these nurses by ensuring they have time to spend with at-risk individuals and advising them about the importance of their role as advocates in care coordination and care planning with these individuals and the healthcare team.

Improving Population Health—Then and Now

During much of her life after returning from the Crimean War, Florence Nightingale was the chief advocate for health in India where British soldiers and natives died for lack of proper sanitation measures. Her statistical analysis and unfailing support of sanitation reforms ultimately resulted in nurses' employment in military hospitals there. These lady superintendents met with Nightingale for advice before departing and carried on a lively correspondence with her during their Indian service. She even sought a medical textbook for one of these nurses, so she could be up to date with healthcare practices (Cook, 1913b).

Today, population health requires a dedicated team approach to improve outcomes for at-risk population groups. Nurses are involved in community assessments to identify health disparities and must engage with other healthcare team members, community partners and stakeholders to develop approaches that work. They are also advocating for these populations with local, regional, and national policymakers and political leaders for regulatory changes that can positively impact population health (Boller, 2017). Today's nurse leaders are excellent resources to develop leadership skills needed by front-line nurses when confronting issues facing at-risk populations. These skills require nurturing and sage advice by nurse leaders to develop fully and make a real difference in people's lives and health.

Reducing Healthcare Costs—Then and Now

Nightingale realized that the costs of poor healthcare were excessive, particularly in her advocacy for improved sanitation in India and the British soldiers there. She shared this with the Marquis of Salisbury, Secretary of State for India. "The man [soldier] is dead or invalided—the man, the most costly article we have; and you have to replace him with another costly article. Is not every neglect or miscalculation on this point sure to add to the national expenditure a far higher amount than would be the capitalized cost of the improvements?" (Cook, 1913b, p. 277).

Her words then are true today as government agencies, organizations, and individuals struggle with cost per capita issues related to insurance access, increasing healthcare costs, large deductibles, and out-of-pocket expenses (Boller, 2017). Value-based care now impacts ambulatory practices as well as hospitals with the goal to increase quality while decreasing costs. Technology advances are designed to reduce per capita costs and increase quality by remote monitoring and telehealth. Nurses focus on health promotion in collaboration with community providers, such as pharmacies and urgent care centers. The focus on behavioral health continues to expand along with community-based care for individuals with chronic diseases (Ma, May, Knotts, & Devito Dabbs, 2018). Nurse leaders can promote cost-effective care by sharing information with their nurse colleagues about value-based care and their role in health promotion.

Improving Provider Work Life—Then and Now (Team Vitality)

Teamwork was different in Nightingale's time. The doctor was in charge of decision-making related to patients and populations. Until Nightingale, trained nurses were nonexistent, and doctors weren't sure how to deal with these newcomers. When she arrived in the Crimea, she was confronted with resistance by some of the doctors, while others welcomed her and her nurses. She was careful to be patient and demonstrate competence and efficiency. She also instructed her nurses to be helpful and only to work in wards where the doctors approved of their presence. It was difficult to develop a team under these circumstances, but she succeeded in the majority of cases. The doctors learned that Nightingale supported them as well as the wounded soldiers and the orderlies, who had ignored the suffering around them, became her greatest allies. Her quiet influence created a team that focused on what was important—the severely wounded soldiers.

Today team-based care is a positive approach to success of the Quadruple Aim. However, team members often work in parallel focused on their own activities in care delivery. This interdisciplinary approach limits team effectiveness. The clinical learning environment requires true inter-professional education and collaboration to achieve positive outcomes for individuals and at-risk populations. This cost-effective approach can help prevent sentinel events by addressing their root causes as a cohesive team that includes the individual client (Chappell, 2016). Today's nurse leaders can educate nurses to actively contribute as members of interprofessional teams and advise them to be learners as well as leaders to ensure team vitality.

What advice do today's nurse leaders have for future nurses in the complex healthcare environment?

- "Listen to your patient and the caregivers. The patient and/or caregivers know when 'something isn't right'—advocate for the patient."—Lya
- "Continue to grow and get education. That is the key to a knowledgeable nurse. Take part in a residency or fellowship—this will create a foundation for you. Seek a mentor who pushes you to be better than you already are in nursing and life. Trust yourself. This is a journey and you should feel joy in caring for patients."—Sheri
- "First 'Get ready for the ride of your life!' Nursing is such a wonderful profession. No matter where you start or think you are going, there are surprises around every corner. I have had wonderful opportunities to care for patients at the bedside, lead quality projects, advocate for health policy at the capital, teach students the importance of professionalism, and volunteer in multiple community groups. The opportunities for nurses are vast! Second, 'Remember the patient is our true North.' As part of the interprofessional team, we are always striving to improve quality, access, outcomes, etc. Certainly, we have the patient in mind when we participate in this work, but we always need the patient perspective. Recently, I was at a quality conference where speakers were presenting on different quality topics and initiatives. The middle of the day was a professional speaker. The

facilitator asked him, 'What advice can you give us on our quality work?' He had been there for all the presentations. His response was 'I really don't care about quality. If I thought for one second that was an issue, I wouldn't have come here. What matters to me is how you treat me and if you really listen to me.' Certainly, this response didn't minimize the quality work we had going on, but it sure did reset our perspective."—Aislynn

- "Look for innovative ways to pursue your passions—nursing isn't confined to inpatient bedside nursing. The profession is vast—find out what you (not your friends or co-workers, *you*) love and unapologetically pursue it. And make sure you take care of yourself emotionally and spiritually. This requires really intentional effort and is especially needed in high acuity areas. Please be proactive about processing and dealing with seeing and participating in trauma at work. Don't tough it out, working under the false assumption that enduring this is your duty simply because you're a nurse. Preventing burnout isn't about taking vacation—it's about learning how to balance being emotionally present with your patients without taking on a great emotional burden every single shift and appreciating work while you're there and home while you're there."—Kati

- "I am going to quote my former dean (when I was an undergraduate at Pitt). Here is what she taught us—I live by it every day—we have a voice and need to actively collaborate and lead in order to ensure that healthcare is the best that it can be! If some procedure is ordered for a patient and you don't agree with it, say so. The days of nurses standing by saying, 'Yes, doctor, of course, doctor, is there anything I can do for you?' is over!"—Jann

- "Listen. Listen to your colleagues, patients and families. Reflect on your learning and share with others."—Kari

- "Never stop learning and never stop helping others learn. In addition: I don't believe in answering questions directly, rather, when I talk with a nurse or student, I say, 'That's a good question. Where do you think you would find that answer?' Then I lead them to policies, procedures; looking at best practices and encouraging critical thinking. 'Never assume' was drilled into me in nursing school and I have never forgotten that."—Cathy

- "*Keep the passion!* Find an area or specialty that you love and do everything you can to stay passionate about the specialty and your contribution as a nurse. *Listen to your patients!* They are the experts about themselves, so listen to their stories. Be their advocate in all situations; at times this will be difficult, but you have to care enough to stand up for them. *Reflect every day!* At a minimum, at the end of your shift each day, do an honest self-reflection on your performance. What did you do well? What did you not do well and why? Ask yourself, 'Am I still passionate about what I do?' If not, or if the passion seems to be weakening, reflect on why the passion is changing and decide on ways to fuel the passion again. You may find you just need to take better care of yourself! Keeping a reflective journal is a wonderful way to self-reflect and plan for continual growth."—Lienne

- "Join a professional organization, start with a BSN."—Andrea
- "If I could offer one bit of advice, it would be this: Nursing has many different avenues, find one that you love. If you love your position, it won't feel like work. Remember, burnout is real. If you find yourself dreading your next shift, please reassess your situation. You may not notice, but your patients will be able to see your unhappiness."—Joseph
- "Be brave … have courage … believe in yourself and your ability, take calculated risks and don't let anyone talk you down. Collaborate with other professions and embrace uncertainty."—Brenda
- "Find what you love to do. There are ample and diverse nursing roles—find which one gives you the most satisfaction and makes it a pleasure to go to work every day. Learn how to be resilient. Share your knowledge with others. Be kind. Be grateful for what you have."—Jean
- "Never give up. Keep pushing through. There will be highs and lows, but at the end of the day it's worth it. We touch lives every single day—regardless of the area/department you work in. Also surround yourself with people who know more than you—that will help you grow and expand into areas you never even imagined!"—Debra
- "Follow your passion. Work where you *want* to be. You will learn all the skills you need if you are excited to go to work. Think bigger than a job. Making a car is a job, being a nurse is a profession, a way of life."—Sue
- "Identify your personal 'brand' and build on your strengths; explore the profession to find a niche where you can make a difference."—Pam
- "Be patient—things don't always happen the way you think they

should, but things have a way of working themselves out and happening when the time is right."—Mary

• "Learning does not stop after you graduate. Continue to read and remain up to date with current practices. Find your passion in nursing, pick a specialty that will make you want to come to work, and share your knowledge. Also join your local, state, and national nurses' association so that your voice will be heard."—Courtney

• "Actively become more than competent in trauma-informed care and nursing skill sets and then become an agent of change in your community. Continually seek out new ways to be and avoid the temptation to treat nursing as a job or vocation but strive to exceed into the realm of professionalism."—Michael

• "Identify your moral compass and stay true to your morals and values."—Dawna

• "Seize the Day! Nursing is the noblest and most trusted of all professions. Embrace the opportunity to promote and protect the health of individuals and the communities you serve. Nursing requires a unique blend of critical thinking, technical ability, empathy, life-long learning, and commitment to give to others. Every day is different, but all days end with a realization that you are making a difference, and someone's world is better because you were there."—Loressa

• "My ivory tower answer is to be sure they are curious, life-long learners, open to opportunities and growth. My practical answer, when I think about it, is much the same. I would say: Find a mentor(s). Be a mentor. Read, write, respond to emails! Ask lots of questions. Be present. Set a goal, reach a goal, repeat. And never, ever, be afraid to ask for help."—Susan

• "Caring for others should not be just a career for you, but rather it should be a way of life. Be a healer to everyone you meet."—Becky

• "Own your practice. Florence recognized we are not just good for cleaning bedpans; we owe it to the theorists that have come before us to continue to advance nursing as a main stakeholder in the medical arena. We need to advance in our professional careers, but not lose sight of the fact that healing happens when we are able to support someone's physical, emotional, and spiritual needs. Never stop being curious about the effect a change in policy or process can have on improving patient outcomes. Speak up and speak often!"—Niki

- "Do not just discard what experienced nurses are trying to share with you, but instead learn from those who have gone before you. You will need to be flexible to overcome the many changes in our profession yet always, always keep the patient first."—Judy
- "Obtain a strong educational foundation, accept opportunities, challenge yourself, and 'lean in' when something needs to be done even if you haven't formally been assigned the work."—Kathy
- "Continually be open to learning the newest technology, skill, device or treatment, but *never* neglect the most important competency: relationship building through communication with patients and co-workers."—Cathleen
- "Our patients need us 24/7. Don't limit yourselves to finding a job that has 'normal' working hours. My proudest and most cherished moments are not those as a leader, but when I was able to be at the bedside with patients and families during their most vulnerable times. When a child could not breathe due to asthma, when a loved one was having an MI, when a spouse of 60 years passed away, when we delivered twins in the backseat of a car outside the ED entrance, and it can go on and on. Don't pass up these opportunities for 'safe' jobs, our hospitals need you more than ever!"—Jacqueline
- "Be flexible, healthcare is consistently changing. That is what makes it exciting. Never stop learning and embrace lifelong learning."—Tina
- "Prepare for lifelong learning, advocacy, leadership, and get your voice on! Find a mentor. I have had the privilege of engaging with amazing mentors throughout the many stages of my career as a student, staff nurse, nursing professional development practitioner, administrator, researcher, writer, presenter, and academic faculty. Nurses and future nurses always need a mentor!"—Charlene
- "Go into the profession for the right reasons; to care for each and every patient and family, to provide hope OR provide comfort, know each day will bring you new opportunities, never stop learning and to never pass up opportunities to grow and try new things—this is what has helped me to steer my career."—Mike
- "Nursing has endless possibilities, spread your wings and see where you land! Most of all, be kind to others and to yourself."—Maureen

This advice from today's nurse leaders reflects determination by nurses to achieve the goals of the Quadruple Aim.

Goal 1. Enhancing the individual's experience of care by listening and learning from him/her and including the individual in the care process. Advocacy for the individual is a nursing responsibility.

Goal 2. Improving population health by being a valued member of the interprofessional team and collaborating with others to serve at-risk populations.

Goal 3. Reducing healthcare costs by demonstrating the worth of education and continuing your own life-long learning to provide cost-effective care.

Goal 4. Improving provider work life (team vitality) by finding joy in your professional life and being passionate about nursing.

This advice is a pathway to success both for nurses and the Quadruple Aim.

9

The Path to Success

"One whose life makes a great difference for all: *all* are better off than if he had not lived; and this betterness is for always, it does not die with him—that is the true estimate of a great LIFE. Live your life while you have it. Life is a splendid gift. There is nothing small in it. For the greatest things grow by God's law out of the smallest. But to live your life, you must discipline it. You must not fritter it away in 'fair purpose, erring act, inconstant will'; but must make your thought, your words, your acts all work to the same end, and that end not self but God. This is what we call CHARACTER."—Florence Nightingale (Cook, 1913b, p. 434)

Nightingale's words reflect praise for one of her colleagues and advice to others. They are also applicable to her own massive success. It is odd putting Florence Nightingale and Ralph Waldo Emerson in the same manuscript, but both would agree that "all great successes are the triumph of persistence" (Emerson, 1803–1882).

Today's nurse leaders have also achieved great success in multiple areas. As they guide their colleagues to achieve the Quadruple Aim, their accomplishments demonstrate multiple aspects of leadership and leadership vital to professional and personal success. Here are their stories.

- "My most significant professional achievement is the accreditation (with distinction) of our transition to practice program. This accreditation validates all the hard work that my team has accomplished for new nurses during their first year of employment. We strive to provide the professional development new nurses need. The greatest validation of that is when the new nurses thank us for our belief in them and our support."—Lya
- "There are so many answers I have for this. If I had to pick one, I would say the recent award nominations I received. I find great pride in lifting up my teams and supporting the great work that

they do. Improving the efficiency of ambulatory practice and ultimately the patient experience has been an honor. This year my boss (the CNO) nominated me for two awards. Two of my colleagues were tasked with collecting stories and feedback and compiling the nominations. I had the opportunity to read what people sent in and have been overwhelmed. The support I have felt from colleagues all around me has been amazing. I have such wonderful comments from physician colleagues, other nurse executives, students I have mentored, community leaders I work with, and even front-line staff. I am humbled by this honor. I am a finalist for the Nightingale Award of (state) in the Nurse Executive Category and am a winner of Top 40 Business Leaders under the age of 40. I know there are specific areas where I make a difference but realizing how far that influence has gone leaves me speechless."—Aislynn

- "I've had some formal achievements (2015 Nurse of the Year) but I think what I am most proud of are those personal emails and messages from new nurses across the world who say my podcast, blog, or book gave them knowledge to take better care of their patient."—Kati

- "I impacted nursing globally by transforming an international association for healthcare educators from one focused solely on continuing medical education (CME) to one supporting interprofessional continuing education (IPCE) across the health professions. I created an interprofessional advisory board, transformed the association's mission from medicine to interprofessional, and developed a new strategic plan. Under my presidency, continuing education professionals engaged in cross-collaboration to disseminate best practices in educational theory, developed national competencies for continuing education professionals, and learned how to implement IPCE."—Jann

- "There are many [achievements]. I feel I have been privileged to work with and learn from great colleagues and to use my expertise to help others. As co-editor of the *Journal for Nurses in Professional Development*, I have had the opportunity to help disseminate research and evidence-based content for our specialty. I especially enjoy mentoring new authors and witnessing their confidence increase as they move through the publishing process. The skills and confidence they gain goes beyond the initial article they publish. Hopefully it establishes a habit of publishing for the rest of their career."—Kari

- "My most significant professional achievement was obtaining my professional certification. It was a way to validate my professional expertise and a matter of pride in my chosen profession and specialty area."—Cathy
- [Most significant professional achievement] "Being part of a network that is modernizing nursing laws and regulations—federal and state."—Andrea
- "I believe accepting a position at the national level has been the most significant achievement. I hope for more to come."—Joseph
- "Since the Magnet program started, I wanted to take a health system to Magnet status since it was exponentially more challenging. I had the opportunity to lead the largest public health system in California to be the first Magnet-designated system in California against all odds and strong union rhetoric against Magnet. All of this while doing my dissertation for my PhD and submitting 17 volumes and 3,571 pages of Magnet documentation."—Brenda
- "Being an ANCC Commissioner for the past seven years. Being part of this group has helped in the design and development of key continuing education and practice transition programs that have impacted the profession of nursing."—Jean
- "Probably getting my PhD. I went back to school twice for graduate work because I wanted a certain job, not because I had a professional career plan. I never imagined I'd be Dr. ... anything, but I'm very proud of the fact that I did. And it positively impacted my kids, three of four are PhDs so they got the message and earlier than their mom. And as I meet new employees, I inquire about their career plans and encourage them to pick big goals. If I can do it, so can they. They like to have someone ask about their future plans and encourage and be excited for them. Get that spark lit."—Sue
- "Guiding the transformation of a national credentialing organization from process to outcomes orientation to emphasize the critical importance of continuing professional development in improving nurses, nursing as a profession, and the provision of nursing care."—Pam
- "Being in a position to influence newer nurses and to help shape the leaders of the future. I get to do this by mentoring students, working with nurse residents, being on the Board of Directors for ANPD and being a mentor for the ANPD Leadership Academy."—Mary

- "Publishing my first article in the *Nurse Practitioner Journal* on 'Identifying Delirium in Older Adults with Pre-Existing Mental Illness.' My dream is to become an author and publish literature that improves the care of adults with mental illness. Although this is my first article, to see part of my dream come true has been truly amazing."—Courtney

- "There are swim lanes to this question. Being selected to serve on the APNA Board of Directors was significant as was receiving the 2014 American Psychiatric Nurses Association National Award for Excellence in Practice: RN. But I have to say that being the lead author of the article 'Engagement as an Element of Safe Inpatient Psychiatric Environments' in the *Journal of the American Psychiatric Nurses Association* is probably the achievement I am most proud of simply because the article admonishes the quality of human to human engagement at the matrix for all care—not just to satisfy TJC or Press-Ganey."—Michael (Michael wishes to recognize his co-authors for their significant contributions to the article)

- "My most significant achievement in assisting nurses in both the U.S. and globally has been participating in elevating the professional role to improve patient care outcomes. Nurses are fundamental to care delivery. If our care delivery can be the 'best it can be' each and every day, we will make a difference in the lives of our patients. From pre-licensure to the doctoral level, I enjoy mentoring and supporting professional growth. We have only just begun to discover the potential of professional nursing."—Dawna

- "Being given the opportunity to lead the ANA Enterprise, the professional organization that represents America's 4 million nurses, whose mission is to 'advance the nursing profession to improve health for all.' As CEO, I can create a vision for the ANA Enterprise that resonates to not only the employees and hundreds of volunteers who do the great work, but also interface and influence others needed to fulfill this mission."—Loressa

- "My most significant professional achievement is also a personal one. My daughter is a registered nurse, and in her I see the reflection of my hard work and endless hours teaching hundreds (thousands?) of nurses and nursing students. Along with her peers, I see a 21st century nurse well prepared with the KSAs to care for patients in an incredibly complex and high-tech world."—Susan

- "Achieving a second master's degree (in nursing education) in the latter years of my professional career."—Becky
- "I am a single parent with a neurologic disease that affects my endurance and physical capabilities. I am proud to be not only a two-year associate nurse but also a bachelor's prepared nurse. At times during both degrees I worked multiple jobs and raised my daughter. A professor once told me that I would never succeed, I needed to go learn to be a qualified medical assistant.... In later years she recognized me as one of the best neuroscience preceptors and mentors there was. I spoke with pride for my profession and myself when I reminded her that she never thought I would succeed. I am proud to serve at the bedside and mentor those entering the field."—Niki
- "My doctorate in nursing is my greatest professional achievement because of the knowledge and skills I learned while pursuing this goal and has allowed me to grow and develop within my profession."—Judy
- "My most significant professional achievement is obtaining my doctoral degree. I went to school while raising two teenagers and working full-time. I changed jobs, accepted a new position as a director of an international credentialing program, and re-built the department. I assumed responsibility for five other credentialing programs including research. My degree provided me with a strong basis for success and the ability to persevere through challenges."—Kathy
- "Developing my teaching skills so that nurses from years earlier can recall lessons learned when they see me today. You can't always tell when you are 'getting through.'"—Cathleen
- "I absolutely loved being part of designing and moving into the Regional Medical Center. We really were creating a hospital of the future; it is an amazing place to practice nursing. I also am proud of being selected and successfully completing the program to be a Magnet Appraiser. For me it is validation of my skills as a nursing leader, plus as an appraiser, I get to visit and learn from other incredible nursing leaders and excellent organizations."—Jacqueline
- "My most significant achievement isn't just one event. When I was a NICU nurse, it was perhaps providing the parent the opportunity to hold their infant for the first time. As a unit-based NPD practitioner, it was watching the orientees evolve and become proficient nurses. As my scope grew, it was creating

programs to develop leaders and watch as they made an impact on their department, organizations, and nursing. This is one of the things I love about nursing. It provides the opportunities to spread your wings, grow and make a difference where ever you land."—Tina

- "My selection as a Fellow in the Academy of Nursing Education was an honor that validated the years of hard work as a nurse educator in practice and academia."—Charlene
- "I don't think I can name one, but I can name many that I am proud of.
  ◊ Receiving my MSN
  ◊ The proverbial ladder I have taken on my career—beginning in 1989 as an Orderly
  ◊ Working for the same organization for nearly 30 years in a variety of roles
  ◊ Overseeing program development—telestroke, telecardiology, new programs at the heart institute—TAVR, LAAO, vascular screenings
  ◊ Watching team members grow and become leaders—both within the heart institute and outside the heart institute. I hope the interactions they had within the heart institute left a footprint on their careers and the decisions they make each and every day."—Mike
- "My current position with the Recognition Program. Everyone I interact with is as passionate about the profession as I am—to be some small part of the work that is done is incredibly gratifying."—Maureen

The achievements of each nurse leader set them on a path to greater success in the future and reflect the importance of education and mentoring for personal and professional advancement. Each has had multiple honors, but their focus continues to be on promoting professional growth for themselves and others These characteristics enable them to lead Quadruple Aim measures successfully in their organizations and serve as role models to other healthcare team members.

10

The Journey Continues

"All great successes are the triumph of persistence."—
Ralph Waldo Emerson

Ralph Waldo Emerson, Florence Nightingale, and today's nurse leaders all have something in common besides the above quote. They have successfully confronted significant challenges in their professional and personal lives to achieve positive results. Today's nurses confront challenges to benefit individuals' perception of care, at-risk populations seeking care, cost efficiency and effectiveness, and team vitality and joy in work. Both nurse leaders and nurses involved in all aspects of care delivery partner with other healthcare professionals to achieve the measures of the IHI Quadruple Aim. Here are the stories of two nurse leaders and how their actions influence achievement of the Quadruple Aim. The subheads were the questions they addressed in the nomination and are from the actual nominating forms.

Aislynn's Story

Nightingale and today's nurse leaders have shared their wisdom in these chapters. One of these leaders was nominated for two awards in the past year: finalist for the Nightingale Award of her state and winner of a state business journal's top 40 business leaders under the age of 40. She was kind enough to share her colleagues' perspectives about her performance in one of her nominations and they validate the contributions she and other nurse leaders achieve as they address the measures of the Quadruple Aim. The following contains quotes from peers and colleagues that demonstrate how Aislyn is a successful nurse leader in achieving all four measures of IHI's Quadruple Aim.

How does this nurse create an environment that is healing and supports empowered professional practice?

"Florence Nightingale was quoted as saying 'never lose an opportunity of urging a practical beginning, however small, for it is wonderful how often in such matters the mustard-seed germinates and roots itself.' I believe Florence would be proud to know that this quote embodies the work of this nominee over the course of an expansive career from a staff nurse to current position in leadership for an academic center."

"In 2016, the health system identified a need for there to be a nurse leader to oversee Ambulatory Care, which led to the creation of a new position: Director of Ambulatory Nursing. This Doctor of Nursing Practice (DNP) became the first in this role and has transformed four distinct divisions; Diabetic Education, Clinical Operations, Clinical Education and Outpatient Care Management. In addition, this nurse leader is the influential, visionary leader for over 500 nurses employed in the Ambulatory Care setting at over 65 clinical practice sites. This DNP has the unique ability to be an extraordinary role model and has successfully unified the outpatient mission to focus on patient/family care by developing the skills of each member on the team. This leader ensures employees are recognized for their outstanding work through weekly nursing executive council announcements, monthly staff meetings, and annual hospital awards."

"All four of this nominee's areas of responsibility have been transformed under this nurse's leadership. One example is in Outpatient Care management. Not long after beginning the role, this nurse identified that while there was a defined Outpatient Care Management team, there were also over 100 other positions in the institution with similar titles reporting through various structures. This DNP created an Ambulatory Case Management forum, uniting the different case managers together to provide a unified voice on their role and responsibilities. This structure allowed nurses throughout the organization to be connected to leadership and provided a forum for standard work and education to be disseminated. RNs who report to this transformational leader describe the applicant as an "excellent communicator, charismatic leader who is willing to take risks and think in alternative ways to achieve the best possible results for patient care and staff satisfaction.

"At this nurse's core is the belief in giving back to the underserved and high-risk populations. This nominee serves on the board of directors for a local free clinic and volunteers there regularly. This clinic provides primary care for individuals who are without health insurance or regular access to care. This nominee has been a vital resource for the clinic who has moved members of the community to awareness and to support the mission of the program. This DNP led a project to raise and allocate funding to install a handicap ramp which increased accessibility for all patients to utilize services at this clinic. This nurse is described by the director as valuing others above themselves no matter their place in society. When gathering information for this submission this was a theme that was echoed by everyone who would describe this nurse leader."

How does this nurse influence quality patient care?

"This nurse influences quality patient care with a comprehensive understanding of what the need is and the expertise to develop and measure meaningful metrics for evaluation of outcomes. Social determinants of health are leading barriers to care and recognized by this nominee as a core patient care value. This nominee has a passion for population-based healthcare that is evident through practice, speaking engagements, and publications. She has gone into the community to interview individuals asking them questions to better understand how they interact with the healthcare system. This nominee is described as having 'a single-minded focus on improving patient-centered clinical outcomes and staff well-being, which they know are inter-related.' The mental model this DNP practices begins with the question 'What is important to the individual and to the staff caring for the patient?' This leader then creates a population-based intervention from this starting point. One notable contribution is the development of an educational video featuring an actual patient about the impact of social factors in that patient's life and health challenges. This nurse utilizes many talents to creatively help learners develop critical thinking skills in the context of real patient problems."

"Historically, this nominee has worked to promote healthcare policy involving healthcare consumers and professionals. This DNP has been an advocate for the nursing profession through working on pieces of legislation for safe staffing and delegation. There have been numerous occasions when this nurse would testify and write comments on nursing related legislation advocating for safe, effective and efficient practice environments. This leader has also had a global impact on patient care with the creation of a state approved, mandatory Child Abuse training program required for RN licensure. This program was taught by this nurse across the state to various professions, including nurses, physicians, social workers, and school workers."

"Healthcare systems have a tendency to work in silos. This DNP understands our healthcare environment is changing and collaboration between systems is needed to provide the best patient care possible. This past spring, this nominee created an Ambulatory Care conference, uniting local health systems together to present on their best practices. This was a time to highlight staff development, care excellence, relationship management, and focus on keeping the patient at the center of all conversations. In writing this recommendation many colleagues were asked to speak on behalf of this nominee. What was striking was how each colleague from varying backgrounds described this DNP as a competent leader, visionary in how this individual is able to create and build teams to provide exceptional patient care through inspirational motivation. The nurse was described as a transformational leader in being able to work with staff to create change with idealized influence. The Chief Operating Officer described her as being a relational-based leader able to make an immediate connection with staff and not only listen, but truly hear staff concerns. Lastly, this nominee was defined as a servant leader in that this person truly puts staff and patients' needs before anything else."

How does this nurse utilize professional standards to advance nursing practice?

"This nominee is a champion and recognized as an expert in developing and implementing professional standards to advance nursing practice.

"The Chief Nursing Officer of our organization gives an example of the exemplary work of this leader: 'This nominee's recent review of the existing Scope and Standards for Ambulatory Nursing Practice determined a need of high importance to revise the internal document to be inclusive of all personnel in the ambulatory healthcare setting, not just nursing. The document was effectively revised, approved and disseminated in an expedited fashion to all of the ambulatory care sites. These changes were required for the electronic medical record and to improve not only safety, but the quality of care for all of our patients.'

"An Associate Chief Medical Officer defines this nurse as an interprofessional discipline leader: 'This leader is creating a supportive environment for the practice of nursing in a diverse and changing workplace; has championed the concept of standard work in the ambulatory practice sites; and helped others to understand why it is essential. This individual is collaborative, thoughtful, engaged, a forward thinker while also taking into account the impact on other professionals, is not trapped in past ways, readily accepts suggestions and critique, and values all members on the team.

"A colleague highlights this nominee's extraordinary work by stating: 'As my preceptor for my graduate program, I observed this leader integrate professional standards throughout our ambulatory care services and throughout the organization. This nominee helped me understand the complex team in the healthcare environment and the need to standardize care expectations. I was also able to observe this nominee in her role as Assistant Professor in both nursing and medical classrooms, highlighting how professional standards provide a foundation of comprehensive collaboration.'

"Finally, the Director of Professional Development for the State Nurses Association highlights this nurse leader's ability to advance nursing practice for the state: 'The nominee is a Commissioner on Accreditation for the American Nurses Credentialing Center since 2016. The nominee collaborates with other nursing healthcare leaders to review and determine accreditation criteria for healthcare organizations in providing continuing nursing education. Through this position, the nominee has been a co-author for publications in the *Journal of Continuing Education in Nursing.* The nominee has been influential at the state governmental level through legislative efforts to improve nursing practice in the state by participating on committees at the state nurses' association and providing an avenue to mentor new nurses and provide leadership and direction for the nurses' association.'

"These four examples showcase how the DNP utilizes clinical expertise and knowledge to integrate professional standards to advance nursing practice. This nurse leader is also a key voice for the nursing profession through scholarship. During 15 years of clinical experience, five posters, five podium presentations, and 10 publications on local, state, national, and international level have been completed along with authoring one book to highlight excellence in nursing care. In addition, this nominee is an adjunct faculty member for four state colleges/universities."

How does this nurse demonstrate positive recruitment and retention strategies/outcomes?

"With the creation of a Director of Ambulatory Nursing, this nominee made it a priority to demonstrate positive recruitment and retention strategies for not only nursing staff, but all ambulatory care staff including medical assistants, technicians, and providers. The results are evident in the outcomes obtained. Within the first months of taking the role, this DNP restructured the Shared Governance Council to include both RN and LPN co-chairs to accurately represent the staff. This leader became an executive sponsor of the LPN Clinical Ladder committee. Within this role, the nominee actively engages with staff to understand their concerns and works to remove barriers to promote quality work environments.

"Through conversations staff shared they felt disconnected from the Nursing Department. This nominee created Ambulatory Nurse Forums bi-annually with the sole purpose to provide dedicated time for informational updates and question/answer sessions with leadership. One topic of the forum was frustration with support for educational opportunities, especially those that were not RNs. The nominee initiated a scholarship program for staff and over the past two years provided more than 10 scholarships for RNs, LPNs, and MAs to attend national conferences.

"The ambulatory care setting includes clinical RN leaders at each site called Senior Attending Nurses (SANs). Prior to this nominee's arrival, a forum was created for this group, but functioned primarily as an informational meeting. This nominee transformed the forum to be a monthly mentoring session. SANs submit topics of interest, and the nominee creates agenda items with expert speakers to address needs. After the initial forums were refocused, the nominee sent out a survey to determine if the forum was meeting the SANs needs. Feedback was they wanted more time to discuss hot topics with each other and ask questions of peers. The forum format was changed, and specific time set aside from each meeting for just this purpose. Many SANs have shared how grateful they are for this forum. One specific SAN said, 'If [this nominee] had not come and taken over the forum, I don't think I would be here. This director is so supportive and helpful. I don't feel like we are alone anymore.'

"The nominee oversees Clinical Education. The department is responsible for onboarding of new clinical staff, and originally consisted of two educators. One educator focused on orientation every month and the other served as a resource to 65 practice sites. Leaders at each site shared concern over the lack of support they had to provide orientation, develop staff professionally, and implement opportunities to retain staff. The nominee strongly believed that more educators were required to support not only the onboarding process, but the entire practice sites. The nominee developed a plan and defended it to senior leadership. Four additional educators were approved and hired. In the first three months, the ambulatory setting had a structured six-month follow-up plan for new clinical hires, an educator for each site to provide professional development, and resources to assist in training for new equipment and/or procedures."

How does this nurse demonstrate effective utilization of resources?

"This leader was tasked with projects upon accepting the position as Director of Ambulatory Nursing. The first priority was to develop and implement a Clinical Operations Division within Ambulatory Care to support the clinical, educational, and research missions of ambulatory care through standard and efficient workflows leading to excellent, accessible, and cost-effective patient care for the communities served. Under this DNP's direction, the Clinical Operations Division collects and utilizes time study data to measure time spent per task in clinic and identify areas of improvement while allowing frontline staff to have a voice in the process. While this nominee trusts the team, they are also a direct resource and guide if an analyst needs assistance.

"Within two years, this group has streamlined processes and created a Standardized Operations Manual. This effort has identified synchronous and asynchronous work of the staff to better identify their tasks and workloads. This DNP led the work associated with this team in addition to advising analysts of fiscally responsible, data-driven ways to request resources. The result was 30 new positions in clinic sites resulting in improved workflow. This result has also improved workplace efficiencies, staff satisfaction and patient outcomes.

"This leader has also empowered the managers to develop the same mindset. This DNP ensures that human resource needs are requested in a fiscally responsible manner. Requests are made on true need and are data-driven and not based on unknown scenarios. Advocacy for staff is one passion for this nominee, especially when it comes to ensuring proper orientation and competency, and there is no problem using resources beyond the walls of the organization to meet those needs.

"One example of an operational and human resource utilization was with the expansion of the diabetic education program within the first six months of hire. Identifying that patients are most at risk when they are transitioning between systems, this nominee partnered with leaders in the medical care of Diabetes to create a transitional Diabetic Educator position that meets with patients in the hospital before discharge and follows up with them at key points after discharge to ensure a seamless transition. The nominee and these leaders have also assessed the need for additional diabetic education services and have begun to standardize the billing process throughout the organization as a way to demonstrate financial stewardship.

"Partnering with a colleague, this leader identified the need to create a Pediatric Case Management structure. They completed a large-scale analysis on the work across the organization to support pediatric care. After the analysis, they felt a new structure was needed, separate from its adult counterparts. Restructuring the pediatric department would align resources, provide clinical oversight, and enhance the patient experience, but had a price tag of $2 million dollars. The structure was presented to senior leadership, return on investment was defended, and the project was approved to move forward" (award application comments, 2018, used with permission).

Michael's Story

Michael is passionate about reducing the teenage suicide rate in the Pacific Northwest by incorporating all four Quadruple Aim measures through innovative approaches. His experience in psychiatric-mental health nursing early in his career demonstrated that members of the healthcare team required education about suicide assessment and prevention to truly inter-vene and steer individuals toward recovery. According to Michael, "Hiding all the dangerous objects, completing periodic assessments, and being kind was not 'care.' I needed a deeper understanding."

As he became active in the American Psychiatric Nurses Association (APNA), ultimately serving on the Board of Directors, Michael sought re-sources to help individuals, populations, and healthcare teams deal with this crisis. His membership in the Association for Nursing Professional Devel-opment (ANPD) also developed his ability to share his message with others.

Michael says, "Oregon suicides have been increasing steadily. Last year they surpassed stroke deaths and continue to exceed deaths by murder, motor vehicle crashes, and breast cancer. While youths are not the highest age group at risk, when a high school student suicides, there is a particularly painful impact on the community. We have had a rash of youth suicides re-cently…. This is not just a hospital issue; it's a community issue."

To create a dialogue with his community, Michael uses a one-hour documentary called *Resilience*. The film describes "the science of Adverse Childhood Experiences (ACEs) and illustrates the cycle of trauma, mental health, and violence" (ANPA, 2019, p. 2). Michael supplements this content with discussions of a panel of local providers about community issues im-pacting suicide rates. These viewings and discussions occur at public loca-tions, including churches and colleges, to engage community members by providing education and awareness to multiple individuals.

Michael also uses his role as President of the Oregon Chapter of the American Foundation for Suicide Prevention to promote Out of Darkness Walks to increase awareness of suicide and remove the stigma associated with the term. His state is the only one where a Walk occurs in a prison and inmates have raised more money than the staff! (APNA, 2019)

Michael is a proponent of the Community Service Delivery Model: Self-Healing Communities, which focuses on avoiding costly duplication of services, providing unified and cost-effective resources, and streamlining activities. The Model focuses on major social problems and use for eight years or more has been shown to reduce suicides by youths (APNA, 2019). He cites the work of the Mid-Valley Suicide Prevention Coalition, which uses a training grant to prepare thousands of laypersons to safely intervene. "I had over 50 people in my class. There is a community demand to be part of the response to this epidemic."

Michael also advocated for a cultural shift in the Level 2 trauma cen-ter facility where he works. It is based on a strategic goal to reduce youth suicides and involves special screenings for teens. "Executive leadership has also implemented a cultural change using the Zero Suicide Academy principles and implementing universal screening in the Emergency Department. As the busiest ED between Seattle and LA, we can make a difference."

Michael's dedication to this issue is resulting in positive change, but his work is not done. As he expresses it: "Yesterday I met with a core group of community health leaders to begin discussions on how to institute a community collective model that would integrate providers' systems, expand community and professional education, and establish a community culture that is trauma-informed.... It's great to see the momentum of a true community response ramp up." It is also the result of one nurse leader's passion to employ Quadruple Aim measures and reduce the incidence of teenage suicide in his local and regional area.

Other nurse leaders profiled here each have their own stories of personal and professional success that significantly contribute to individuals' perception of care, improving the health of at-risk populations, reducing per capita costs of healthcare, and promoting team vitality and joy in work. Each nurse leader pursues positive results as Nightingale did so successfully over a century ago. Their success is truly the triumph of persistence!

11

Population Health
Goals and Considerations for the Future

"She was born at Florence on May 12, 1820, in the Villa Colombaia, near the Porta Romana, as a memorial-tablet now affixed to the house records."—Cook, 1913a, p. 4

The 200th anniversary of Florence Nightingale's birth is in 2020. Her achievements continue today in the work of nurse leaders to advance healthcare and the Quadruple Aim. At the start of a new decade, it's time to examine successes and challenges in achieving each of these measures as we explore the future of healthcare in the United States. Beginning with a review of national and regional initiatives, we will examine the future role of nurse leaders in each Quadruple Aim measure.

Population Health—National Quality Forum

In 1999, the President's Advisory Commission on Consumer Protection and Quality in the Healthcare Industry determined that an organization was essential to support and safeguard the protection of patient populations and healthcare quality via measurement and public reporting The resulting National Quality Forum (NQF) is designated by the Office of Management and Budget as the sole consensus-based healthcare organization in the United States. This status makes healthcare practices and measures endorsed by NQF as evidence-based best practices to improve care to multiple populations. Currently, nearly 300 of these measures are used in over 20 federal pay-for-performance and public reporting programs, state programs, and private-sector programs. The National Quality Forum also guides the Department of Health and Human Services (HHS) to use the best available measures in performance-based payment, public reporting and other programs based on input of multi-stakeholder groups in both the public and private sectors (National Quality Forum, n.d.).

This process began when the Patient Protection and Affordable Care Act established a National Quality Strategy in 2011 as a national effort to improve healthcare delivery, patient outcomes, and population health. Collaboration between private and public stakeholders is essential in aligning quality improvement activities and quality measures. This fit what was then known as the IHI Triple Aim framework—improving the individual's experience of care, improving population health, and reducing per-capita healthcare cost. The National Quality Strategy was a three-pronged approach that included (1) Better Care—patient-centered, accessible, safe, and reliable care; (2) Affordable Care—reduced healthcare costs for individuals/families, employers, and the government; and (3) the Healthy People/Healthy Communities initiative—improved population health through performance measures that address social, environmental, and behavioral elements of health. The National Quality Forum was the logical choice to coordinate stakeholders' quality improvements and disseminate them via HHS federal healthcare programs that impact significant populations (Wilson & Leavens, 2015).

The National Quality Forum (NQF) created the Measure Applications Partnership (MAP) within the Patient Protection and Affordable Care Act to establish multi-stakeholder groups that collaborate to (1) determine best-available performance measures; (2) provide sound input on measures for HHS; and (3) promote affiliation of performance measurement within the private- and public-sectors. This collaboration is truly unique and "balances the interests of consumers, businesses and purchasers, labor, health plans, clinicians and providers, communities and states, and suppliers" (National Quality Forum, n.d.).

MAP advances healthcare priorities nationally by selecting performance measures that help federal programs achieve transparency, improvement, and value for everyone. This process includes reviewing available NQF-endorsed performance measures that have evolved from a rigorous evaluation by multiple stakeholders to ensure that these measures address important aspects of care, provide reliable information, and compare results for providers and agencies. NQF only endorses quality measures that meet strict criteria. These include (1) outcomes measures that determine if desired results were achieved; (2) composite measures that combine multiple individual measures into one performance measure; (3) episode of care measures that use a patient-centered framework to address patient outcomes over time; (4) healthcare disparities measures that use a set of disparities-sensitive measures to address cultural competency; (5) standardized measures that reduce duplication of results; (6) measures for patients with multiple chronic conditions using a framework to support quality of care for these individuals; and (7) eMeasures and health information technology using electronic data to capture performance. The NQF endorsement process requires consensus by multiple stakeholders and NQF's role is to facilitate improvement measures by these stakeholders, rather than developing its own measures (National Quality Forum, n.d.).

Population Health Framework Project

In 2014, the NQF drafted its first Community Action Guide as part of a three-year HHS-funded project to help communities begin or improve population health programs. Projected to save over $19 million over ten years based on existing programs to improve health and wellness in U.S., populations, the NQF created the Guide to help communities work with local healthcare providers and public health agencies to increase population health programs nationally. The Action Guide included (1) definitions of terms, (2) 10 elements essential to achieve lasting improvements in population health, (3) recommendations and ideas for actions, and (4) examples of tools, measures, and other practical resources. The 10 elements required

1. self-assessment about readiness to participate;
2. leadership in organizations and within the region;
3. organizational priority-setting and planning process;
4. community health assessment and process for asset mapping;
5. prioritized and agreed upon set of health improvement activities;
6. selection and use of performance targets and measures;
7. strategic communication that is audience-specific;
8. joint reporting on progress toward achieving results;
9. scalability indications; and
10. plan for sustainability [Wilson & Leavens, 2015].

Ten diverse groups were selected geographically to field test the Action Guide 1.0 based on an environmental scan of conceptual frameworks on national, state, and local levels. The charge for each selected group was to provide implementation input that would refine the Action Guide and validate its applicability to their current or planned population health improvement projects. The story of one of the selected groups illustrates the impact of the Guide on a regional level (National Quality Forum, n.d.).

Regional Action—Michigan Health Improvement Alliance (MiHIA) and Population Health

The Michigan Health Improvement Alliance (MiHIA) based in mid-central Michigan is a formal, multi-stakeholder, 501(c)(3) non-profit community collaboration, established in 2007, working to achieve a community of health excellence for the 14-county region it serves in central Michigan. MiHIA's mission is fulfilled by focusing on the Quadruple Aim and to serve as the regional hub for sharing health information and collaboration among all sectors, including patients and their families. By producing a call to action across multiple programs and organizations, their goal is for their region to become a national leader and a model for health that leads to a positive economic impact.

Functionally and operationally, MiHIA works at many levels. In some cases, MiHIA acts as the convener for multiple parties, establishing shared goals and objectives, setting collective targets, or aligning business plans. In other cases, MiHIA is an assessor, evaluating processes and offerings to reduce redundancies, conducting environmental scans, or providing health data. MiHIA also seeks funding to bring resources to the area and facilitates or supports projects or initiatives that will impact better health and healthcare in the region.

In 2010, MiHIA was chosen as a participant in the Triple Aim Framework focusing on health optimization in area communities. In 2014, ten MiHIA counties ranked in the lower 50 percent of national *County Health Rankings* for many of the indicators including physical inactivity, tobacco use, and obesity. Realizing that untreated obesity and continued smoking lead to costly chronic illnesses, decreased population health, and increased costs, MiHIA focused on chronic disease prevention and up-stream interventions to improve population health. They also set a goal to improve their *County Health Rankings* that all 14 counties were in the top two percentiles (Michigan Health Improvement Alliance, n.d.).

MiHIA was selected by the National Quality Forum to participate in the development of Guide 1.0, which included information about root causes of obesity and actions to take to address causes by implementing options for physical activity. The Guide 1.0 also provided information about tobacco use prevention as well as how to develop a plan for sustainability "to continue operating, funding the work, and remain productive over time" (National Quality Forum, 2014, p. 34). MiHIA used the resources in the Action Guide by influencing numerous assets essential for their ongoing work, "such as convening power, and engaged Board, passionate participants, a comprehensive health dashboard, and a strong track record of success" (National Quality Forum, 2014, p. 41). Their collaboration with the National Quality Strategy and the NQF extended through development of the Community Action Guide 2.0 and 3.0 by sharing their experiences to refine the information. MiHIA's Population Health Strategy Team based their strategic plan on additional goals that also focused directly on obesity and physical activity (Michigan Health Improvement Alliance, n.d.). In addition to the areas described above, the strategic plan included two priority areas where MiHIA can best improve population health in the region. These areas are (1) creating opportunities and regional resources for all communities to address modification of health behavior and (2) improving access throughout the region "to primary, dental and behavioral healthcare" (Michigan Health Improvement Alliance, n.d.). The MiHIA Population Strategy Team used Dashboard 4.0 and standardized methodology and process in their 2018 Regional Community Health Needs Assessment (RCHNA). They thoroughly analyzed the results and developed the Regional Community Health Improvement (RCHIP) to address these two top regional health priorities (Michigan Health Improvement Alliance, 2019).

Current Status

At present, only four of the 14 counties served by MiHIA have been ranked in the top two quartiles (range 1–42) of the *County Health Rankings*. Half of all counties in the region range between 36–68, with a median value of 54. Six counties are still in the fourth quartile (range 64–83). The mean score for all 14 counties is 54, placing them near the middle of all 83 counties. Work continues to address smoking, obesity, inactivity, and food choices/food deserts. However, this goal is unmet and has been revised to read, "By 2024, all 14 counties in the MiHIA region will be ranked in the top 2 quartiles of the *County Health* Rankings" (Michigan Health Improvement Alliance, 2019).

Additional goals related to this macro strategy show mixed results.

1. By 2024, decreasing the percentage of adults age 20-plus who are obese (BMI≥30) to 33 percent is also not met with obesity rates increasing from 33.5 percent in March 2015 to 34.7 percent in March 2019.

2. By 2014, decreasing the percentage of adults age 20-plus reporting physical inactivity to 23 percent is showing progress toward the goal with rates decreasing from 26 percent in March 2015 to 24.9 percent in March 2019.

3. By 2024, increasing individuals who report access to exercise

opportunities to 80 percent has increased from 60.2 percent in March 2015 to 70.6 percent in March 2019 [Michigan Health Improvement Alliance, 2019].

Their sustainability continues to make them a regional leader as they pursue complex changes to address these population-specific goals (Michigan Health Improvement Alliance, n.d.).

The Future of Population Health

What will happen as we move into a new decade? The Patient Protection and Affordable Care Act may or may not continue to exist in the future, but some of its tenets must remain. The National Quality Strategy and the work of the National Quality Forum on consensus-based best practices to improve care to multiple populations arose from the Patient Protection and Affordable Care Act and must continue to evolve even if the Act itself does not. This book is not a platform for a particular healthcare system in the United States. It is focused on how the Quadruple Aim will progress (or not) in 2020 and beyond. Population health is a difficult concept to quantify. There is no one definition or description of population because it differs depending on how the individuals within it are classified (e.g., diabetics, geographic demographics, elders, religious groups, at-risk youths, adults with congestive heart failure, enrolled insurance populations, etc.). Each population has different needs—physical, mental, spiritual, social, and economic— and meeting these needs and expectations is a monumental task even if they are clearly defined and uniform in nature. Unfortunately, improving population health is seldom (if ever) that simple.

This is why some of the side benefits of the Patient Protection and Affordable Care Act, like the National Quality Strategy and the work of the National Quality Forum must continue to exist and thrive. Both of these involve public and private stakeholders and strive to align evidence-based quality improvement activities and quality measures (Wilson & Leavens, 2015). This work is critical if the quality of life and health is to improve for diverse populations. This will be a lengthy and complex process. The work to date is a beginning, but we have not done a deep dive into all complex health needs of multiple populations.

Additional support must identify these populations and ascertain their diverse health needs. Two populations with the same diagnosis will have differing health needs. One size does not fit all. This will make addressing and improving health in these populations a complex challenge. Groups like the Michigan Health Improvement Alliance will be essential in the coming decade to impact population health issues on the regional level. Although progress will be slow and at times absent, these regional groups must be supported by national groups as well as stakeholders in local communities. They need to focus on small wins and strategies that will make a positive difference in their areas. A network of support among these groups will keep their eye on the goal of improving the health of the communities they serve. These groups and the National Quality Forum realize that multiple public and private stakeholders must be actively involved to move the dial on population health. It is frustrating struggling to meet goals that would benefit people in these regions. Education is a good starting point, but it is not enough alone to change behaviors that have been ingrained for many years. The desire to change must be present and not everyone in a population group has a desire to change. It is vital for everyone trying to impact population health to understand that simply telling people why they should change their behavior will not result in 100 percent success. MiHIA and other groups have tried multiple avenues to advocate for health improvement (e.g., smoking cessation classes, walking paths, exercise programs, community gardens, etc.) (Michigan Health Improvement Alliance, n.d.). These groups must be flexible as population needs and expectations shift to fulfill their mission and vision in practice. Areas that do not have an effective regional health improvement team will need to establish one that includes individuals from the populations they will serve as well as multiple public and private stakeholders with a sincere desire to improve health and quality of life in their region. MiHIA and other existing groups must share their knowledge about what works and what can be improved with their new colleagues. The National Quality Forum has initiated some of this collaboration with the test groups for their Action Guides. They can serve as a national resource bringing teams together to study and implement evidence-based best practices in their regions.

Health care improvement measures can no longer occur in silos. To eventually succeed, everyone must collaborate, and everyone's ideas must be valued.

Nurse Leaders and Population Health

Nightingale's Influence

Florence Nightingale set an example for nurse leaders to follow in her interactions with multiple Commissions and Parliament to address population health issues during the latter half of the 19th century. Her leadership impacted the people of India through collaboration and communication with providers there as well as seeking legislative relief for public health. In the words of her biographer, "Miss Nightingale's private letters and printed articles did something to fill the gap. She had the ear of the great personages; they knew how much she knew, and they respected her devotion and sincerity. They listened to her, and her letters often produced the kind of stimulating result that sometimes follows a parliamentary intervention" (Cook, 1913b, p. 281). Her influence was described by the following written exchange by a supporter in India: "The result is just what I expected," wrote another Anglo-Indian, on the occasion of a later intervention by Nightingale. "They treat me with contempt, but they don't ignore you. The first thing the Governor did on seeing your letter was to sit down and write a full exoneration of himself to the Secretary of State. The second, I have no doubt, will be to call for his officials and hurry on the work" (Cook, 1913b, p. 281).

Population Health—Nurse Leaders 2020 and Beyond

The next decade will not be easy and nurse leaders must be part of the solution in addressing the health needs of multiple populations. Nurses are leading interprofessional teams and sharing their knowledge with other team members as well as the populations these teams serve. They also realize that needs and perceptions of population members are not uniform. Clients who have congestive heart failure have different backgrounds, knowledge, and willingness/unwillingness to change behavior. Nurse practitioners are often the health provider for this population who must address the need for behavioral change to improve health. It is vital to take the time to learn about the members of at-risk populations to better understand their expectations and lack of compliance with care. All populations are not homogeneous. And life experiences play a significant role in how a population member deals with health changes. Working with the population group may be very different from working with individual members. One of our nurse leaders shared how she became involved in Alzheimer's causes, prevention, and screening, even advocating at the Federal level by testifying to Congress about the importance of research for this at-risk population. Her story is powerful because it shows how nurses can lead in population health. Nursing education continues to evolve as advanced practice nurses grow and practice. Nursing influence at the regional, state, and national level is also vital and many state nurses' associations as well as the American Nurses Association are educating nurse leaders to talk with their legislators about health needs of at-risk populations they serve. Their voice when used is powerful and can make positive changes to advance population health. Nurse leaders, regardless of title, have a message that others don't. They just need to articulate it backed up by evidence to those who can initiate beneficial healthcare changes. More nurses are running for office and winning to advocate for those in need. In the next decade, nurse leaders will continue to speak out and serve on boards, including regional and community groups like MiHIA. Using Nightingale as a role model, their presence and voice are essential to solving issues impacting population groups.

12

Improving the Individual Experience of Care

Future Implications

> "I was sick in hospital at Balaclava and she nursed me through a long illness of Crimean fever. She was with me, I might almost say, night and day, and it is to her good nursing and energetic attention I owe my recovery. Previous to my illness I had had experience of her friendship when at Scutari, where the hospitals were crammed with dead and dying, and cholera was carrying off hundreds of victims a day; it was amid such scenes as this that I constantly beheld Miss Nightingale."—Surgeon-Major Vincent Ambler, June 1883 (Cook, 1913b, p. 334)

This tribute by a former patient demonstrated how Florence Nightingale improved the experience of care by her presence in the Crimean War. The individual's experience of care today occurs in multiple settings but must be positive regardless of outcome.

Improving the Individual Experience of Care— National Quality Strategy

The National Quality Strategy has six priorities designed to improve health and healthcare quality for individuals and the community in which they live. These six priorities are (1) person and family-centered care; (2) patient safety; (3) effective communications and care coordination; (4) health and well-being; (5) affordable care; and (6) prevention and treatment of leading causes of morbidity and mortality (Wilson & Leavens, 2015). Within this initiative are three aims: (1) healthy people; (2) better care; and (3) affordable care. These aims are dedicated to ensuring that the individual achieves improved health and healthcare quality that he/she can afford (Wilson & Leavens, 2015). Starting with the three aims, this section will discuss healthy people and better care. The next Quadruple Aim measure will discuss affordable care.

Healthy People

Healthy People/Healthy Communities is a reflection of the Healthy People framework developed through collaboration of the Department of Health and Human Services (HHS), other federal agencies, public stakeholders, and the Secretary's 12-member Advisory Committee on National Health Promotion and Disease Prevention composed of national public health experts. Healthy People has existed since the Surgeon General's report in 1979 titled *Healthy People: The Surgeon General's Report on Health Promotion and Disease Prevention*. That report initiated 10-year national initiatives to improve the well-being and health of people in the United States. Its goals are designed to (1) help people achieve longer, high-quality lives; (2) improve groups' health by removing inequalities and attaining health fairness (equity); (3) promote good health for everyone by creating positive physical and social environments; and (4) promote healthy behaviors, development, and quality of life in all life stages (Healthy People 2020, n.d.).

Objectives are evidence-based, measurable, and ambitious to achieve health promotion and disease prevention during a 10-year period of time. Data collection from multiple sources enables Healthy People leaders to monitor progress and establish goals for each succeeding decade. Healthy People 2020 selected 26 Leading Health Indicators (LHIs) from its objectives to address high-priority health issues. Of these, 14 of 26 LHIs have demonstrated improvement or met their target. Four indicators—Air Quality Index, exposure of children to secondhand smoke, homicides, and adults meeting Federal guidelines for muscle strengthening and aerobic physical activity—have met their targets. Another 10 indicators have improved including adult screening for colorectal cancer, hypertensive adults with controlled blood pressure, children receiving recommended vaccines, injury deaths, infant deaths, total preterm live births, HIV-positive persons' knowledge of serostatus, percent of students receiving a high school diploma four years after beginning ninth grade, reduction in adolescents using illicit drugs or alcohol, and reduction in adult cigarette smoking. Although these indicators are not met, they are moving toward their targets. Three indicators have worsened—suicide, adolescents with major depressive episodes, and individuals who have seen a dentist in the past year. One indicator—reproductive health services for sexually experienced females in the past 12 months—only has baseline data available at this time (Healthy People 2020, 2014, pp. 3–4).

These 2020 indicators and their results will be used to inform Healthy People 2030. Data and feedback on progress must be shared with the public as well as Federal and public health agencies. Although behavioral change is achievable with concerted effort, the United States trails other developed countries on key indicators for well-being and health, such as infant mortality, obesity, and life expectancy. Healthy People is determined to help individuals, as well as populations, achieve its vision—"a society in which all people live long, healthy lives" (Healthy People 2020, n.d.).

Better Care

The National Quality Strategy as described by the National Quality Forum defines Better Care as "improve overall quality, by making healthcare more patient-centered, reliable, accessible, and safe" (Wilson & Leavens, 2015, p. 3). Healthy People 2020 assesses this indicator as Access to Health Services, but only looks at the percent of individuals under 65 years with medical insurance with a target of 100 percent (baseline 83.2 percent in 2008 and 83.1 percent in 2012) and the percent of individuals with a primary care provider with a target of 83.9 percent (baseline 76.3 percent in 2007 and 77.3 percent in 2011) (Healthy People 2020, 2014, p. 3).

Improving the Individual Experience of Care— The Leapfrog Group

The individual's experience with access to care that is safe and reliable requires a look at a national organization that is a driving force for quality and safety in healthcare—The Leapfrog Group. In 1998, a group of business leaders met for dinner and discussed the dysfunctional U.S. healthcare system. As employers, they spent significant funds on healthcare without being able to assess quality or offer employees choices for plan selection. In 1999, the Institute of Medicine report "To Err is Human" disclosed that preventable medical errors in hospitals resulted in nearly 98,000 deaths annually. Over 60 business leaders partnered with the Robert Wood Johnson Foundation, the Commonwealth Fund, and the Business Roundtable to finance a new approach to individual care that evolved into the Leapfrog Group. The name denotes progress by taking giant leaps forward to initiate changes that can impact significant numbers of people (leapfroggroup.org, n.d.). Since its inception in 2000, the national, non-profit Leapfrog Group has made significant inroads in quality of care and patient safety.

Realizing that transparency is essential in evaluating healthcare performance, the Leapfrog Group began its work with three initial "Leaps"—ICU physician staffing, computerized physician order entry, and evidence-based hospital referral—using seven Regional Rollouts to survey 496 targeted hospitals nationally. Within a year, the number of hospitals had nearly doubled, and Leapfrog began its public reporting website to encourage transparency in reporting data. By 2003, the original three "Leaps" were increased to include the National Quality Forum's Safe Practices for Better Healthcare on Leapfrog's hospital survey. The Health Plan Users Group began in 2004 to evaluate the efforts of health plans to include Leapfrog data in their tools for members, tier levels, and pay for performance programs. The Leapfrog Group realized that healthcare purchasers needed help to identify the highest-value hospitals locally, regionally, and nationally. In 2005, Leapfrog created the Leapfrog Hospital Recognition Program to provide this support for employers, health plans, and large healthcare purchasers. Seven Regional Rollouts had expanded to 31 by 2006 enabling Leapfrog to target over 50 percent of U.S. hospitals. That year, the Leapfrog Group designated its first Top Hospitals (leapfroggroup.org, n.d.).

In 2007, the Leapfrog Never Events Policy was published and a question about the policy was added to the Leapfrog Hospital Survey. This resulted in 52 percent of hospitals adhering to the policy and CMS publicly announced decision to not pay for eight types of Never Events beginning in October 2008. Leapfrog became a force for patient safety and quality in healthcare. In 2008, an initial "Leap"—computerized physician order entry (CPOE)—resulted in a CPOE Evaluation Tool for hospitals. By 2009, Leapfrog began its first Top Rural Hospitals Awards and a year later the Top Hospitals of the Decade were recognized (leapfroggroup.org, n.d.).

Leapfrog data continued to produce momentous results that impacted patient safety nationally as illustrated in the following example. When the Leapfrog data on early elective deliveries showed that thousands of elective deliveries were scheduled too early for infant safety, a national call to action resulted (2011). By 2014, in partnership with the March of Dimes and Childbirth Connection, Leapfrog reported a significant decline in early elective deliveries and the national rate decreased from 17 percent in 2010 to 4.6 percent in 2013 and 2.8 percent in 2015. Leapfrog's focus on maternal and neonatal health continued in 2015 when the organization released the first national standardized cesarean section rates by hospital (leapfroggroup.org, n.d.).

Leapfrog continues to lead the way for patient safety and quality of care by awarding letter grades for hospitals based on how safe they are for the patients they serve (2012). The Leapfrog survey process continues to expand to provide employers, insurers, and most of all consumers with the ability to make informed decisions about healthcare. Surveys include the Leapfrog Hospital Survey (voluntarily completed by over 2,000 hospitals annually) and the Leapfrog Ambulatory Surgery Center Survey (new voluntary quality and safety survey with data collection from April 1–November 30, 2019), The Leapfrog Hospital Safety Grade evaluates over 2,600 hospitals annually on their ability to keep patients safe. The program is voluntary and free of charge to participating hospitals and uses national performance measures in alignment with The Joint Commission, the Centers for Disease Control, and Centers for Medicare and Medicaid Services (leapfroggroup.org, n.d.).

Leapfrog has implemented a Value-Based Purchasing (VBP) Program where participating hospitals can benchmark their performance against others and Survey Results give each participating hospital an overall Value Score. This Value Score ranks hospitals and establishes financial incentives or rewards for those with highest scores. The Survey performance results for all participating hospitals is compiled in a report that each hospital receives biannually. The Leapfrog VPB Program is unique and can be implemented rapidly. The results are transparent and create an effective payment method that stimulates additional improvements. This unique program was designed with scientific rigor by a panel of experts—researchers, academic faculty, employer representatives, and health economists based on a standardized set of evidence-based measures. Hospitals are benchmarked locally, regionally, within health networks, and nationally. The Leapfrog Hospital Survey serves as the single source of data enabling hospitals to implement the program easily. Transparent results encourage conversation between purchasers of healthcare and hospital leaders to establish specific improvement goals. Domain scores are based on key performance elements including

1. maternity care (used in CMS Inpatient Quality Reporting [IQR] Program and Value-Based Purchasing [VBP] Program and aligned with The Joint Commission [TJC] and National Quality Forum [NQF]);
2. medication safety (aligned with National Quality Forum Safe Practice);
3. hospital-acquired conditions (used in CMS Inpatient Quality Reporting [CMS IQR], VBP, and Hospital Acquired Conditions Reduction Programs and aligned with NQF and CDC/National Healthcare Safety Network [NHSN]);

4. inpatient care management (used in CMS IQR Program and aligned with NQF Safe Practice); and

5. high-risk surgeries (used in CMS VBP Program) [leapfroggroup. org, n.d. and cms.gov, 2018].

Leapfrog results are also publicly reported to assist individuals seeking the highest-value care and making informed decisions to improve their healthcare experience (leapfroggroup.org, n.d.).

Regional Action—MiHIA and Improving the Individual Experience of Care

The Michigan Health Improvement Alliance (MiHIA) continues to use metrics and data-driven measures to assess regional progress in patient experience and quality of care. The organization has set high targets and looks at success based on the following goal: "Health systems in the MiHIA region will strive to obtain the highest possible Hospital Safety Grade [Leapfrog]" (MiHIA.org, 2018, p. 4). MiHIA influences the progress in access to comprehensive primary care, treatment effectiveness, and appropriate hospital utilization through multiple initiatives. These initiatives include (MiHIA. org, 2018, p. 4):

- Centering Pregnancy;
- Choosing Wisely;
- Dashboard 4.0;
- Healthier and Happier Families;
- Perinatal Quality Collaborative;
- Pharmacists and Barriers to Care;
- Regional Opioid Strategy; and
- THRIVE Initiative

Current Status of Initiatives

Centering Pregnancy

Centering Pregnancy is a program designed to improve prenatal care using a group setting. Women with similar due dates are assigned to groups of eight to 10 that are led by an experienced facilitator. The structured process occurs in a comfortable setting and uses health assessments, interactive learning, and increased time and attention from healthcare providers to support better health behaviors resulting in better outcomes. Expectant mothers attend ten two-hour sessions during their pregnancy and have 10 percent additional time with their care provider. The opportunity for interaction with peers creates friendships that would not have been possible without the program. Sessions focus on a variety of topics including (1) labor and delivery process; (2) breastfeeding benefits; (3) nutrition counseling; (4) managing stress and common pregnancy discomforts; (5) importance of good dental care/hygiene; and (6) significance of post-delivery care. Centering Pregnancy promotes self-confidence, self-care, patient-centered care, friendship and support, increased time with the provider, and better health outcomes (Michigan Health Improvement Alliance, n.d.).

According to 2018 data, 149 pregnant women from 8 counties in the region attended group prenatal care by Centering Pregnancy. There were 29 Centering Pregnancy groups resulting in 69 percent of participants initiating breastfeeding compared to 53 percent of pregnant women using traditional care. Only 25 percent of participants had another pregnancy within two years compared to 37 percent of traditional care participants (MiHIA. org, 2018, p. 6).

Choosing Wisely

The Choosing Wisely Campaign began in 2012 as an initiative of the American Board of Internal Medicine to help physicians and individuals make effective and smart healthcare choices by decreasing overuse of procedures and tests. Choosing wisely encourages conversation between the individual and the provider about relevant care and treatment. Unnecessary testing may be harmful, and individuals need to learn what is appropriate for their health issues. There is now a list of tests or procedures that should be discussed prior to ordering. Individuals seeking healthcare also should ask five questions before any test, procedure, or treatment.

1. Do I really need this procedure or test?
2. What are the side effects and risks?
3. Are there safer, simpler options?
4. What happens if I don't do anything?
5. What is the cost and is it covered by insurance?

Forty-seven percent of physicians in the region state that patients ask for unnecessary procedures and tests at least weekly. However, Choosing Wisely enables individuals to ask the right questions during their appointments to make informed decisions about their care. Its guidance includes materials outlining recommendations about applicable tests and treatments. Communication and collaboration between individuals and providers are essential to make sound healthcare choices (Michigan Health Improvement Alliance, n.d.).

Based on 2018 data, the Choosing Wisely Campaign involves 1,700 healthcare providers and 20-plus community partners in the MiHIA region (MiHIA.org, 2018, p. 6).

Health Dashboard 4.0

In 2009, MiHIA developed a health dashboard to provide a centralized data source for healthcare consumers, providers, and professionals. The Health Dashboard graphically describes a snapshot of current status and key indicators' historical trends to enable users to make informed decisions. It is an electronic tool for information about healthcare performance with the objective of improving the quality of life and health status for the 14-county region it represents (Michigan Health Improvement Alliance, n.d.).

Health Dashboard 4.0 (2017) is the latest update to the web-based data information system which assists health systems, health departments, communities, providers, and consumers to improve health outcomes and performance. The Dashboard provides users with access to over 2,300 indicators based on 400 data sources, advanced analysis, over 2,100 best-practice strategies correlated with regional health issues, customized reports, and a user-friendly website. The Dashboard benefits individuals by helping them understand their community's health issues and providing access to programs that positively impact their quality of life and well-being. Numerous foundations, universities, healthcare organizations, health plans, and health departments support the MiHIA Health Dashboard 4.0 as a single data resource for individuals to quickly locate pertinent information. The site is updated as changes occur on a monthly or annual basis and its indicators are based on both state and national sources (Michigan Health Improvement Alliance, 2019).

Based on 2018 data, Health Dashboard 4.0 has 21 organizations as partners, uses over 300 indicators from 30 sources, and has resulted in 2,100 promising practices (MiHIA.org, 2018, p. 6).

Healthier and Happier Families

The "Healthier & Happier Families: Preventing and Fighting Childhood Obesity" program is a partnership between MiHIA and Kurbo Health to reduce obesity and diabetes in children ages five to 19 years who live in a 14-county region of central Michigan. Kurbo Health began in 2013 and is a mobile, research-based coaching program licensed by the Pediatric Weight Control System of Stanford University. Kurbo coaches help children and families lose weight and learn healthy eating habits using a mobile application and weekly coaching sessions. The application enables families to track exercise and food while engaging with videos, games, and challenges to learn proper nutrition. It uses a Traffic Light Diet system by Dr. Leonard Epstein to arrange foods into greens, yellows, and reds. Users learn to understand food choices and slowly decrease the number of reds (unhealthy foods). Kurbo coaches conduct live weekly coaching sessions for 15 minutes via phone, text or video (Kurbo.com, n.d.).

This 12-week program has been used by over 50 children and families within 6 regional counties since 2017 with no charge for participation. It is capable of serving up to 400 children and families. Based on 2018 data, children have experienced an average reduction of 2.83 percent in Body Mass Index and have lost an average of 11.81 pounds. Currently this initiative has over 20 community partners (MiHIA.org, 2018, p. 29).

The Regional Diabetes Prevention Program (DPP) which began in 2015 is also being implemented to help address chronic diseases. Its purpose is to prevent or delay the onset of Type 2 diabetes among pre-diabetic individuals in central Michigan. The program is one year long with 16 weekly core sessions and six to eight monthly post-core sessions where participants learn about incorporating physical activity and healthy eating into their daily lives. MiHIA and its partners increased awareness of prediabetes and diabetes prevention programs and aligned the Regional DPP with state and national agencies. MiHIA's greatest achievement has been leading regional partners to participate in the Medicare Diabetes Prevention Program, resulting in DPP as a covered benefit for Medicare beneficiaries. In 2018, 498 individuals were enrolled in the MiHIA regional DPP grant program. Four counties have had 37 sessions since April 2015 and 13 new Lifestyle Coaches were trained by MiHIA in 2018. This brings the total number of trained Lifestyle Coaches to 52 with three regional Master Coaches. Participants have achieved a 5.2 percent weight loss and added 305 average minutes of physical activity (MiHIA.org, 2018, p. 26).

Perinatal Quality Collaborative

MiHIA, in partnership with the Michigan Department of Health and Human Services and the Saginaw County Mental Health Authority, are co-leading the development of the Prosperity Region 5 Perinatal Care System Quality Improvement Initiative. The Steering Committee is composed of multiple stakeholders who are implementing strategies to ensure that mothers and babies thrive and are healthy resulting in positive health outcomes. Centering Pregnancy has already been implemented and was described in a previous section. Other focus areas include (1) early entry into prenatal care; (2) perinatal substance abuse; (3) Neonatal Abstinence Syndrome (NAS); (4) screening for adverse childhood experiences; and (5) cultural competency. The Collaborative seeks prevention with use of evidence-based practices to improve maternal and infant health. Baseline data showed that an average of 25.5 percent of pregnant women in Prosperity Region 5 smoked while pregnant compared to 16 percent for all of Michigan (2016). The NAS rate in Prosperity Region 5 was 568.13 per 100,000 live births compared to the state range of 315.23–157.56 per 100,000 live births. Statistics for 5,829 births in Region 5 showed that 9 percent were preterm, 1.3 percent were very low birth weight, and 8.5 percent were low birth weight deliveries (MiHIA.org, 2018, p. 32).

Pharmacists and Barriers to Patient Care

MiHIA held focus groups to recognize the role of community pharmacists in enhancing adult engagement and adherence to medication regimens, including medication self-management. Pharmacists and physicians met with social workers and mid-level health providers to (1) expand collaborative practice agreements to improve patient care services and outcomes; (2) recommend systems designs to optimize positive outcomes; (3) review current activities of healthcare teams related to medication therapy and patient care models; and (4) collect data for use by the State of Michigan to increase patient involvement in hypertension treatment (MiHIA.org, 2018, p. 30).

These focus groups were followed by a panel discussion of pharmacists and physicians in May 2019 that discussed how pharmacy services can improve quality and health outcomes. Panel participants described best-practice models where pharmacists' involvement in managing chronic conditions improved medication use and care management. It was an opportunity for healthcare providers to seek collaboration with local pharmacists and a chance for pharmacists to explore how to expand their services (Michigan Health Improvement Alliance, n.d.).

Regional Opioid Strategy

MiHIA's 14-county region has also been hit by the opioid epidemic. In 2016 MiHIA identified a need to have a multi-strategy, multi-sector approach to addressing the epidemic. They stepped in to play a leading role in combatting this crisis by coordinating efforts to develop a Regional Opioid Priority Strategy Map. A Workgroup was formed and has representatives of more than 30 organizations in the region that include subject matter experts, healthcare professionals, public health organizations, community organizations, behavioral health organizations, law enforcement officials, and universities. The Opioid Strategy Map tracks comprehensive strategies, activities and interventions used in the region.

The template, on the following page, is available as an open source template and is backed by a rich set of information and tools at via the Opioid Coalition Resource Hub. *www.insightformation.com/ocrh* (used with permission).

This resource is located on Health Dashboard 4.0 and enables MiHIA to provide information within the region that enables providers to prevent duplication of services and share best practices with each other. The tool identifies needs, gaps, and barriers in service. Users can find innovative approaches used by communities across the nation that would be applicable in the region (MiHIA.org, 2018, pp. 19–20). The Regional Strategy Map continues to be a work in progress with ongoing collection of data from multiple sources that inventory current regional approaches and activities (MiHIA.org, 2018).

In August 2018, a community coalition accelerator workshop focused on sharing ideas, tools, and techniques in priority focus areas. Community partners learned about additional techniques and resources to augment their approach in creating a future comprehensive community strategy (MiHIA.org, 2018). There are currently 39 unique partner organizations in the Opioid Priority Strategy Work Group who focus on prevention of opioid abuse and misuse via education, policy, diversion prevention, and alternative clinical interventions. Teams develop 60- and 180-day goals to address selected strategies using evidence-based interventions in six priority areas: (1) enhancing peer recovery groups; (2) expanding and improving risk factor screening and Screening, Brief Intervention, and Referral to Treatment (SBIRT); (3) improving protective factors for youth; (4) Medication Assisted Treatment (MAT); (5) non-opioid/non-pharma treatment; and (6) reducing occurrence and impact of Neonatal Abstinence Syndrome (NAS) (MiHIA.org, 2018).

Some of these six strategies have made progress while others are still in the planning stage. (MiHIA.org, 2018).

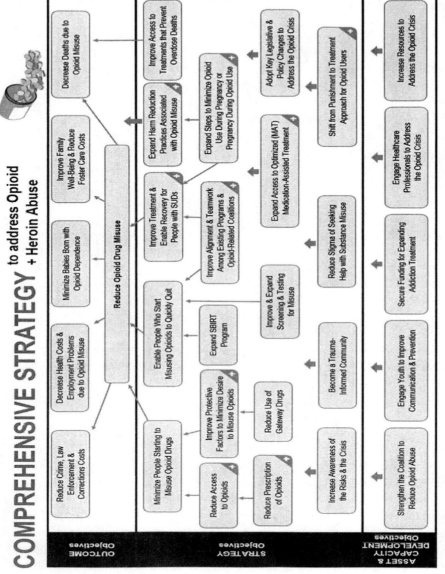

THRIVE Initiative

The final initiative is THRIVE (Transforming Health Regionally in a Vibrant Economy). This is a multifaceted approach to address both poor health outcomes and poor economic outcomes in the Great Lakes Bay

Region and is a collaboration between MiHIA and the Great Lakes Bay Regional Alliance (GLBRA). The initiative began in 2017 and has finalized a 34 intervention Portfolio focused on job creation, regional attractiveness, addressing the social determinants of health, healthier living, improved care for physical illness, and improved mental healthcare. Each of these directly impacts individuals in the region who need access to basic health services and advanced specialties. Other aspects of THRIVE relate to economic and cost of care issues and will be discussed in the next chapter along with the Bridging for Health initiative.

Improving the Individual Experience of Care in the Next Decade

Healthy People 2020 will soon be replaced by Healthy People 2030. Its goals have expanded to emphasize well-being, health literacy, and economic environments that promote health. There also is a new Goal: "Engage leadership, key constituents, and the public across multiple sectors to take action and design policies that improve the health and well-being of all" (Healthy People 2030 Framework, 2019, p. 2).

As we enter a new decade, increased focus on individual health and well-being is essential to reduce unnecessary utilization of health services while ensuring a high quality of life for every individual. As we have seen, governmental, national, and regional agencies strive to improve quality of care for individuals. However, such organizations cannot achieve success without the support and knowledge of the individuals they serve. Health literacy is essential. Education is a good starting point, but alone it is not enough to make a positive difference. The individual must also assume responsibility for his/her own health and attaining the knowledge to achieve the highest quality of health and well-being.

The Leapfrog Group provides user-friendly data that enables individuals to make sound decisions about their healthcare (leapfroggroup.org, n.d.). This is a vital resource that many individuals either are unaware of or don't access. There must be a concerted effort to disseminate such information nationally to those who ultimately will benefit. Community health centers and health providers must educate their clients about how to access such resources and how to interpret their results.

Organizations like MiHIA have promoted increased time spent with health providers in their Centering Pregnancy Program and have achieved positive benefits (Michigan Health Improvement Alliance, n.d.). Such an approach would help other individuals, particularly those with chronic health conditions to interact with peers and gain valuable time in face-to-face discussion with their providers. Providers must use pertinent questions and conversation to establish patient understanding about health issues, treatment, and care options. Using the teach-back method is a way to determine the individual's degree of health literacy (Health Literacy Universal Precautions Toolkit, 2nd edition, 2015). Teach-back validates understanding by asking the individual to restate in his/her own words the information given. It can also include a Show Me aspect to reinforce medication administration, dosage, and technique. The provider may say, "We've talked about your Insulin administration. Show me how you will do that, how much you will give and when." Eliciting "yes"/"no" answers will not verify the individual's knowledge and understanding. This opportunity for dialog is beneficial to the individual's health and the relationship between provider and patient (Health Literacy Universal Precautions Toolkit, 2nd edition, 2015).

The individual must be an active participant in his/her own care and willing to ask questions and clarify understanding. The healthcare team must keep the individual at the center of care and advocate for his/her needs. Information must be provided in language the individual can understand and restate. Health and well-being apply to everyone and national, regional, and local groups must collaborate to ensure that all individuals attain the mission of Healthy People 2030 to "promote, strengthen, and evaluate the nation's efforts to improve the health and well-being of all" (Healthy People 2030 Framework, 2019, p. 3).

Nurse Leaders and Improving the Individual Experience of Care

Nightingale's Influence

Florence Nightingale knew the importance of families to the soldiers she cared for in Scutari. Women camp-followers often followed their husbands and loved ones to war and their situation was deplorable. Many were in rags and malnourished. She assigned the wife of a military chaplain to care for these women. When they were able to seek employment, she had boilers put in a Turkish house where wives washed bedding in hot water for the comfort of wounded soldiers (Cook, 1913a, pp. 195, 197).

Nightingale's concern with the health of individuals and families continued after her return and in 1892, Nightingale began a new initiative in villages around her Claydon home in Buckinghamshire. She saw a need for education in health of local villagers and spearheaded the creation of sanitary instruction by the District Health Officer and a team of "health-missioners" trained to share practical information with villagers for their better health and well-being. Her hands-on approach increased villagers' knowledge of hygienic practices (Cook, 1913b, pp. 383–384). This instruction was not a panacea but marked a beginning for rural sanitation in England.

Improving the Individual Experience of Care— Nurse Leaders 2020 and Beyond

Nurse leaders will play a pivotal role in improving the individual experience of care and his/her health and well-being. To achieve success, we need to explore a historical perspective that is applicable today.

In the early 20th century, Lillian Wald advanced Nightingale's work providing care in partnership with others to address issues beyond physical care that impacted entire families in New York slum neighborhoods. She mobilized community resources, as organizations like MiHIA are doing today. Wald's emphasis on cleanliness, healthy food sources, and education for children and families parallels the use of strategy maps discussed previously (MiHIA.org, 2018).

Wald's visiting nurse model put nurses and social workers at the crossroads of medical care and individuals in the community who need healthcare services. When the Sheppard-Towner Act was passed in 1921, public health nurses expanded their work on health promotion and prevention of maternal and infant mortality. Today, public health nursing does not realize the vision of Lillian Wald as funding sources, physicians, and healthcare facilities have not fully supported this model as it was designed (Pittman, 2019). This presents an opportunity for the future as care for individuals expands to include greater emphasis on prevention and education to support health and well-being. Nurse leaders must support interprofessional collaboration with the individual and significant other(s) at the center of care. Social determinants of health will continue to be a focus of Healthy-People 2030 because these social, economic, and physical conditions occur in individuals' environments and impact health and well-being. Based on HealthyPeople 2020 data:

- 74 percent of children ages 0–17 years live with at least one parent employed full-time year-round (2014);
- 66.7 percent of high school graduates enrolled in college by the next October (2017);
- 12.3 percent of persons in the U.S. live in poverty (2017);

- 17.5 percent of children ages 0–17 years live in poverty (2017);
- 34.2 percent of households spend more than 30 percent of income on housing (2012);
- 65.4 percent of households earning less than 200 percent of the poverty threshold spend more than 30 percent of income on housing (2013);
- 16.2 percent of all households spend more than 50 percent of income on housing (2013);
- 24.2 percent of renter households spend more than 50 percent of income on housing (2013);
- 6.9 percent of children ages 0–17 years have lived with a parent who has served time in jail or prison (2011–2012);
- 70.3 percent of persons eligible to vote are registered to vote (2016); and
- 61.4 percent of persons eligible to vote report voting in the most recent November election (2016) [HealthyPeople2020].

While some of these indicators have improved, work remains on affordable, safe housing, economic and educational opportunities, community-based resources, and access to health services (HealthyPeople2020). Nurses are uniquely positioned to fulfill Wald's holistic focus on individuals as members of families, communities, and workplaces that affect their physical and psychosocial well-being. The nurse leaders profiled here understand that and practice with the individual at the center of care in their decision-making. As the number of nurse practitioners evolves and their practice environments move into community settings, they must address four core functions to create a framework for change in multiple settings. These nurse leaders must

1. establish a climate of trust with individuals, families, and communities by demonstrating compassion and support;
2. conduct an in-depth assessment of an individual's health, family dynamics, and community factors;
3. develop partnerships with multiple community stakeholders in addition to health professionals; and
4. expand focus to address disparities and gaps in health outcomes that require collective solutions [Pittman, 2019].

One of our nurse leaders put it best when she said that nurses are the key to healthcare reform. They must develop their power and use it to benefit the individuals, families, and communities they serve.

13

Reducing Per Capita Cost of Healthcare Without Compromising Quality

"These are the ABCs of the reform required. (A) So long as a sick man, woman, or child is considered *administratively* to be a pauper to be repressed, and not a fellow-creature to be nursed into health, so long will these most shameful disclosures have to be made. The past system of mixing up all kinds of poor in workhouses will never be submitted to in the future. The very first thing wanted is classification and separation. (B) Uniformity of system is absolutely necessary, both for efficiency and for economy. (C) For the purpose of providing suitable establishments for the care and treatment of the Sick, Insane, etc., consolidation and a General Rate are essential. The entire Medical Relief of London should be under one central management which would know where vacant beds were to be found, and be able so to distribute the Sick, etc., as to use all the establishments in the most economical way."—Florence Nightingale on Poor Law Reform, 1866 (Cook, 1913b, pp. 133–134)

Reducing Per Capita Cost of Healthcare: Healthcare Reform

This quote shows that healthcare reform is not a new concept. There is agreement that healthcare must be accessible, high quality, and cost effective, but there is no one single path to achieving these results. There are numerous players and stakeholders in this journey, including providers, insurance carriers, healthcare facilities, communities, businesses and payers, individuals with pre-existing conditions, and at-risk populations. There is also no magic bullet that works for everyone. This chapter will explore the history in the United States of healthcare reform, current status and challenges, and future implications for organizations, populations, and individuals nonjudgmentally.

Healthcare reform began with Theodore Roosevelt in 1912 when he advocated for healthcare for all after his term of office ended. When that effort failed, healthcare reform languished until President Roosevelt developed Social Security, but didn't include coverage for medical services in the legislation. President Truman wanted a health system but couldn't generate the votes to pass any legislation. President Johnson achieved the most progress toward healthcare reform by passage of the Medicare and Medicaid programs in 1965. President Nixon advocated expansion of health coverage via employers, individuals, and private insurance. He was unable to pass any legislation before leaving office in 1974. President Clinton tried to revamp the healthcare system but didn't succeed. However, national discussion ensued about healthcare that resulted in expansion of insurance coverage to more individuals, resulting in the Patient Protection and Affordable Care Act of 2010 (Agarwal, 2019 & ObamaCareFacts.com, 2018).

In addition to improving access to care, the Act was designed to reduce taxpayer costs for healthcare by including the Triple (now Quadruple) Aim. Accountable care organizations discussed previously experimented with cost-reduction measures. Health insurance exchanges were developed for small businesses and individuals to buy coverage with subsidies for those below 400 percent of the poverty rate. Medicaid was expanded to cover low-income individuals up to 133 percent of the federal poverty level. (ObamaCareFacts.com, 2018) Everyone was to maintain health insurance or face a penalty (since rescinded as unconstitutional). Court cases are currently pending to determine the constitutionality of the Law itself.

Prior to the 2016 election, the Council of Accountable Physician Practices, an affiliate of the American Medical Group Foundation, issued an executive summary to encourage candidates to (1) increase movement to value-based care, (2) advocate use of health information technology, and (3) improve quality measurement and reporting to identify providers and systems achieving the best clinical outcomes (CAPP, 2017).

With this background information, the Department of Health and Human Services (HHS) is the federal agency responsible for promoting affordable healthcare in the United States. Its Strategic Plan begins with a strategic goal to "Reform, Strengthen, and Modernize the Nation's Healthcare System" (HHS.gov, 2018). Three divisions—CMS, AHRQ, and FDA—are responsible for implementing programs to "promote affordable healthcare, while balancing spending on premiums, deductibles, and out-of-pocket costs" (HHS.gov, 2018). Even though 91.2 percent of U.S. citizens had health insurance or medical assistance for all or part of 2016, government-sponsored plans paid for health services for 37.3 percent of these individuals. Health spending nationally is expected to rise at an average rate of 5.5 percent per year from 2017 to 2026. Government healthcare spending will be greater than other payers as Medicare enrollment rises and if subsidies continue for low-income participants in health insurance exchanges (uncertain at this time). The United States spends more per capita for healthcare than other Organization for Economic Co-operation and Development (OECD) countries, but health outcomes are not always better as a result of this spending (HHS.gov, 2018).

Health and Human Services (HHS) is focused on ensuring healthcare costs for citizens at affordable levels and minimizing healthcare spending by the government. HHS and its partners plan to achieve these results by making consumers more informed, developing options at lower costs, innovative service delivery and payment models, and promoting competition in the healthcare marketplace and preventive care. HHS is working with States to help them provide affordable, competitive insurance plans that will best meet their citizens' needs. HHS has ways to pay incentives to physicians and other healthcare providers who care for Medicare beneficiaries and provides alternative payment models that can be used to reward value rather than volume for an episode of care, a clinical condition, or a population. HHS also evaluates alternative payment models that involve multiple stakeholders and seek to reduce costs and improve quality of care. The Agency shares this data and evidence from innovative models with policymakers at both Federal and State levels to demonstrate methods that work to "reduce healthcare costs and improve quality" (CMS.gov, 2018).

The Department of Health and Human Services and its divisions use multiple strategies to reduce healthcare expenditures nationally. These measures include

1. support appropriate use of lower-cost, high-quality providers (e.g., community organizations, community health personnel, etc.);
2. advocate discharging patients to home and community-based settings at site-neutral payment rates to promote post-acute care efficiency and coordination;
3. increase access to affordable, safe, high quality generic medications by expediting access to lower-cost alternatives and enhancing competition for prescription drugs;
4. use educational campaigns to promote the value of generic drugs to payers;

5. offer outpatient medications at reduced prices to eligible health-care organizations through the 340B Drug Pricing Program;

6. supply data on causes, prevalence, and consequences of high financial costs for healthcare, including social determinants that increase costs;

7. partner with organizations and States to teach consumers about options for health coverage and how to identify the best plan for themselves;

8. inform consumers how they can access and use their benefits;

9. monitor trends in health insurance plans re premiums, deductibles, and out-of-pocket expenses/maximums;

10. review regulatory requirements that may unfairly affect some providers; and

11. promote preventive care to reduce future medical costs [HHS.gov, 2018].

Health and Human Services (HHS) also wants consumers to make informed decisions about their healthcare and seeks transparency about the value and cost of healthcare with health literacy tools, models, and websites comparing options, services, and treatments, such as Hospital Compare and Nursing Home Compare. HHS realizes that reduction of premium increases will require more younger, healthier consumers to buy plans and stabilize the market. The Agency seeks to streamline enrollment and eligibility processes in the community so every population can access needed services. Value-based programs incentivize providers for quality and value, not volume. These programs strive to lower overall cost of care and HHS advocates increasing the percentage of Medicare payments and funds used by alternative payment models (HHS.gov, 2018). This is an ambitious agenda that will require significant time and resources to accomplish.

One example is an innovative payment model launched by HHS in 2019. This model for emergency ambulance services creates new incentives and is value-based to ensure that patients receive the right care, from the right provider, in the right setting, and at the right price. The model enables ambulance staff to provide care on site or with telehealth and uses alternative sites (e.g., primary care offices, urgent care clinics, etc.) to meet Medicare beneficiaries' needs more effectively and efficiently. The model is scheduled to start in early 2020 and will include two payment options—one for on-scene treatment and another for transport of Medicare beneficiaries to alternate destinations when ED care is not required. Ambulance suppliers and providers will earn up to a 5 percent payment adjustment in the later years for the five-year trial period based on their attainment of key quality measures. The model will also encourage implementation of triage lines for low-acuity 911 calls (HHS.gov, 2018). This is one example of planning by HHS for future cost-effective measures in care delivery.

Reducing Per Capita Cost of Healthcare— Regional Initiatives

Regional backbone organizations realize that excessive costs result in many individuals and at-risk populations not seeking out healthcare or complying with medication and treatment regimens. In the Great Lakes Bay Region, healthcare, like many other communities in the United States, accounts for almost 20 percent of the economy and the region's economic success must be integrated with cost effective, quality healthcare. The Michigan Healthcare Improvement Alliance's THRIVE (Transforming Health Regionally in a Vibrant Economy) initiative was introduced in the last chapter and recognizes that economic success and health and well-being are inextricably linked. In collaboration with the Great Lakes Bay Regional Alliance (GLBRA), MiHIA is co-leading this initiative to build a stronger regional comprehensive strategy. THRIVE's focus on continued economic growth and excellent health outcomes is foundational and has attracted notice from thought leaders in both Michigan and nationally. MiHIA and GLBRA each bring essential elements for success. GLBRA's mission is "regional growth and vitality" (MiHIA.org, 2019). MiHIA has an established track record of successful commitment to regional health and a network of relationships with health industry leaders. Together they have created a multi-year action plan that fosters engagement by multiple stakeholders to achieve and sustain health and economic outcomes. Each of these outcomes is interdependent and are achieved through 34 interventions. Both organizations have engaged community leaders, regional organizations, educational institutions, and healthcare professionals to collaborate and position THRIVE to build a stronger economy that will advance healthcare. The region has distinct advantages for success. Communities are strong and cohesive and there are plentiful resources available to address medical and health needs. However, many programs addressing health disparities are siloed and lack a unified approach. THRIVE uses a comprehensive master plan where all stakeholders combine their efforts to strengthen the economy and improve the health of the communities in the region (MiHIA.org, 2018).

THRIVE's robust and thoughtful strategic planning has led to an implementation pathway. The process began in the summer of 2017 when 80-plus stakeholders were interviewed to seek ideas about economic and health improvement, discuss local viewpoints, and look at possible challenges and opportunities. That fall, system mapping identified five priority areas for concurrent economic and health improvements. Priority Teams assigned to each of the five priority areas spent the winter/spring of 2018 gathering evidence-based interventions and establishing metrics. These interventions were assessed based on strategic alignment, capacity of implementation, and cost effectiveness. In partnership with ReThink Health, the THRIVE Portfolio was tested via a simulation model and analysis "to project impact and expected outcomes on numerous metrics over a twenty-year horizon" (MiHIA, GLBRA & ReThink Health, 2019). The portfolio was finalized in the fall of 2018 and leaders in the region collaborated to obtain capacity-support funding for three years. The Steering Team convened with representation from healthy systems, employers, the medical school, and other key economic stakeholders to launch the THRIVE Portfolio and continues to coordinate the initiative and measure its progress. Plans include phasing of interventions, creating a financing strategy, incorporating multiple funding sources, and overseeing effective communication.

To list a few outcomes, economic impact will be measured by (1) regional job increases for new and current employers, (2) reduction in working-age residents leaving the region, and (3) residents' economic prosperity (MiHIA.org., 2018). ALL THRIVE's Top 5 Strategic Priorities are

1. developing provider capacity through health education and profession pathway;
2. increasing preventive care and well-being, including mental healthcare;
3. reducing barriers to social determinants of health through community involvement;
4. advancing attractiveness of the region related to care access, cost, quality, and delivery; and
5. creating jobs in the region [MiHIA.org, 2019].

Another initiative that was mentioned in the previous chapter looks at aligning financing and funding sources to improve population health and reduce per capita cost of healthcare. Bridging for Health: Improving Community Health Through Innovations in Financing is sponsored by the Robert Wood Johnson Foundation (RWJF) and links collaboration, financing, and health equity. MiHIA partnered with Bridging for Health to determine what funding tool or tools will finance programs that improve health outcomes. MiHIA selected a Health and Well-Being Fund to include multiple funding sources in a pool that is held to support wellness prevention and interventions to improve health outcomes. This innovative approach blends financial resources that can fund activities which individual organizations couldn't achieve alone (MiHIA.org, 2018).

A Health and Well-Being Fund is not a standard funding plan for projects. It uses models to develop regional commitment and capacity for ongoing sustainability. The Fund is a multi-year strategy that includes a shared commitment and infrastructure. This collective focus enables stakeholders to address preventable challenges to health and well-being. Investments are distributed based on their collective impact. The Fund also encourages investment by diverse funding sources and foundations to enhance impact (MiHIA.org, 2018).

MiHIA will use a three-prong strategy for the Health and Well-Being Fund called a Three Generation Approach. This approach builds funding and investments that support a preventive care portfolio for the region that will address needs and gaps. Generation I establishes the core fund and strategy for targeted intervention by delivering a Virtual Diabetes Prevention Program in all 14 counties that addresses reduced BMI, A1C, blood pressure, absenteeism and cost of care while increasing physical activity, productivity, and self-esteem. Generation II expands prevention strategies by investing and adding additional financing and funding sources. Generation II focuses on portfolio expansion for preventive care, mental health, and well-being initiatives. Generation III increases regional funding and multi-sector engagement/involvement using the THRIVE initiative previously discussed (MiHIA.org, 2018).

The Importance of Reducing Per Capita Cost of Health Care

Federal agencies and employers are trying to rein in healthcare costs. The National Quality Strategy selected affordable care as one of its three aims. The Leapfrog Group was founded on the premise that transparency would help people make informed decisions about care and employers and purchasers should only pay for the best outcomes at the best price (Wilson & Leavens, 2015, and leapfroggroup, n.d.). Although these programs are helpful, they are not a panacea for cost per capita reduction in healthcare. Prescription costs continue to escalate and health insurance is no guarantee that all or most healthcare expenses will be covered. Some experts believe universal coverage is the answer and others believe free market forces will prevail. Regardless of the outcome, individuals must be advocates for their own health and well-being. That includes making healthy nutritional choices, increased activity, knowledge about medications—dosage, purpose, side effects, and how to take—as well as preventive care options. Individuals, especially those with chronic conditions, must actively participate in their own care. This means asking questions and seeking clarification. Community agencies will help if contacted, but every person must be accountable for his/her own health and well-being. Using clinics rather than emergency departments if indicated will reduce use of expensive resources and escalating medical costs.

Physicians and other providers must reach out to individuals with co-morbidities to prevent exacerbations and ensure that they are stable. A follow-up call from offices at regular intervals may catch problems before they become complex. Support groups for at-risk populations should be encouraged as a way of connecting with peers and for early surveillance that can reduce inpatient stays and costs. Use of non-physician providers can also reduce per capita costs if the provider is knowledgeable and can refer to advanced care as needed.

Value-based payments will continue in the future and bundled payments for specific disease conditions must be explored. Health information technology and quality measurement and reporting can increase efficiency and standardize quality measures for payers (CAPP, 2017).

Controlling medication prices is currently difficult to achieve and insurance plans vary in payment options. These areas will require support from agencies like Health and Human Services and legislators to develop a strategy that will reimburse these companies at a reasonable rate and protect the rights of consumers at the same time. That's a tall order, but health equity won't be achieved without a resolution.

Regional organizations, like the Michigan Health Improvement Alliance, are working to improve health and well-being, including access, programs for individuals and at-risk populations, and reducing costs by tying health to economic vitality. Their work must be replicated nationally and national discussion must ensue about what healthcare reform should be in the United States and how meaningful outcomes can be achieved.

Nurse Leaders and Reducing the Per Capita Cost of Healthcare

Nightingale's Influence

This chapter began with a quote from Florence Nightingale about need for healthcare reform in London. The sick poor were housed in workhouse infirmaries in terrible conditions under the Poor Law. When Nightingale made her proposal for reform, the Whigs were being replaced by the Tories who were reluctant to make any changes. She outlined her proposal to a committee appointed by the new government and mobilized the press to enflame public opinion. Her efforts resulted in the Act of 1867, which was the foundation for improvement in the Poor Law. A single district was created in London to treat the sick instead of housing them in workhouses. The "Metropolitan Common Poor Fund" was created and charged with maintaining the facilities, medicines, and schooling of pauper children. "Miss Nightingale counted up the gains, and said, 'This is a beginning; we shall get more in time" (Cook, 1913b, p. 139). According to her biographer: "The Act of 1867 was the foundation on which many improvements in medical relief under the Poor Law have been laid, and the principles implied in the Act—the separation of the sick from the paupers, and in the case of London the making medical relief a common charge—are likely to receive yet further recognition. They are the principles for which Miss Nightingale contended. Her influence in forming the public opinion which made the legislation of 1867 possible was referred to in both Houses of Parliament" (Cook, 1913b, p 39). Her prophecy was fulfilled in later years as nursing care in workhouses under Nightingale nurses led health reform

Reducing Per Capita Cost of Healthcare: Nurse Leaders 2020 and Beyond

Regardless of their role or title, all the nurse leaders profiled in this book clearly understand that cost effectiveness and efficiency are essential to ensure that individuals receive high-quality care at reasonable cost. Some work with patients in hospitals and community health settings. Others lead in public and private agencies and organizations. Some educate students, nurses, and other healthcare providers about the relationship between cost and quality. All seek to streamline processes and systems that will benefit those they serve and reduce per capita costs of healthcare.

Nurse leaders in the next decade must continue these activities and encourage other nurses to really listen to patients, especially those who have been non-compliant with treatments or medications. If the individual has to choose between lodging or food and taking an expensive drug, resources must be mobilized to assist the person with social determinants of health. Nurse leaders must know how to contact available resources and collaborate with others to address the person's needs. This doesn't mean that the nurse leader has all the answers. Sometimes just asking questions will lead to a positive response. When working with at-risk low-income populations, a resource file can help providers seek financial support for these individuals from available agencies.

Since the current political climate is unsettled, nurse leaders must learn how to interact with legislators about fiscal funding that impacts care delivery. Nurse leaders must advocate for individuals who cannot advocate for themselves to ensure their health and well-being.

Another approach involves a new nursing role as coaches. A nurse coach uses a holistic approach to interview individuals about their health behaviors, current health status, and goals for health and well-being. Health insurance providers now support health coaching for their enrollees to improve their health and reduce costs for the providers. Value-based care is designed to keep people healthy and attain shared risk payer contracts where health facilities assume more patient costs and reimbursement is based on value, not volume. Nurse coaches in these settings can achieve the best outcomes for providers, payers, and individuals. As individuals pay more out-of-pocket costs for their healthcare, nurse coaches can help them reduce these costs. Nurse coaching is a recognized specialty with two available certifications and training programs endorsed by the American Holistic Nurses Association. This role continues to evolve as individuals and other stakeholders seek positive clinical outcomes and sustained health and well-being that will reduce costs for everyone (Knutson, 2019).

14

Improving Provider Work Life (Team Vitality)

Where Do We Go from Here?

> She was constant in seeing that her "daughters" took proper holidays; sometimes helping to defray the expense, more often having them to stay with her in South Street or in the country. She was constant, too, in sending them presents of books—both of a professional kind likely to be of help to them in their work, and such as would encourage a taste for general literature.—Cook, 1913b, p. 258

> Miss Nightingale put a high value too, upon *spirit de corps* as an aid to maintaining a high standard of duty ... all the Sisters who went out into the world from the [Nightingale] School were encouraged to regard themselves as members still of a corporate body, however widely separated from one another they might be ... each was inspired to take courage from the success of others.—Cook, 1913b, p. 259

These quotes show that improving provider work life is not a new concept, but it has taken on new meaning recently as the 4th Quadruple Aim. In Nightingale's time, teams were highly structured with physicians at the head. Today, team leadership varies depending on the situation and other health providers and individuals seeking care are actively included in decision-making. Burnout and compassion fatigue are newer terms that adversely affect team functioning and the health and well-being of team members.

How to Improve Provider Work Life (Team Vitality)

Fortunately, other terms—resilience and mindfulness—positively affect the team and its members' performance. Resilience is "ability to face

149

adverse situations, remain focused, and continue to be optimistic for the future" (Kester & Wei, 2018, p. 42). Mindfulness is "awareness of the present moment" (Penque, 2019, p. 40) and helps individuals "separate from negativity and gain insight into the situation" (Penque, 2019, p. 43).

In 2017, ANA Enterprise initiated a national initiative to improve health in the United States by enhancing the health of registered nurses. According to then-American Nurses Association (ANA) President, Pamela Cipriano, "*Healthy Nurse, Healthy Nation* is a grand challenge intended to make major social change in the country. We believe that by improving the health of nurses, we will improve the health of the nation. That's a long-term, audacious goal" (ANA Enterprise, 2018, p. 30). Healthy Nurse, Healthy Nation (HNHN) focused on five indicators for nurses and nursing students to improve their own health and enable them to serve as role models for others. The five indicators are nutrition, sleep, physical activity, safety, and quality of life. Participants join the HNHN Connect web platform and take a health-risk appraisal. Each person has a profile page where he/she has access to blogs, resources, discussion groups, challenges, and makes a commitment for health improvement. Participants become part of an online community to support each other in attaining positive health goals. HNHN engaged over 25,000 participants and attracted over 350 partners from multiple organizations and stakeholders. Survey results at one year are based on over 9,000 participant responses and collated to address each of the five indicators (ANA Enterprise, 2018, p. 30).

Nutrition

Programs like Simply to Go encourage more intake of fruits and vegetables Survey results showed that only 14 percent of participants eat recommended fruit and vegetable daily servings. Only 24 percent eat recommended daily servings of whole grains. Although 54 percent noted that healthy options are available at work, 55 percent found these more expensive than other items. The average Body Mass Index (BMI) of these survey participants was 28.8, which is greater than a normal BMI of 18.5–24.9 (ANA Enterprise, 2018, p. 35).

Sleep

Tips and suggestions to improve rest and sleep included setting a sleep goal, limiting caffeine and shutting off electronics before bedtime, and using ear plugs, darkening shades, white noise, or relaxing sounds. Survey results showed that 14 percent of participants fell asleep or nodded off in the past

30 days while driving and most of these were nurses between 26 and 32 years of age (ANA Enterprise, 2018, p. 34).

Physical Activity

Challenges like Step It Up, walking groups, using steps, and parking further away from destinations helped increase physical activity for some participants. At one year, (1) about 40 percent used exercise facilities; (2) 45 percent never participated in vigorous activity; (3) 19 percent didn't participate in weekly light or moderate aerobic activity; and (4) younger nurses commonly participated six to 10 times a week in about 30 minutes of moderate exercise (ANA Enterprise, 2018, p. 33).

Safety

Survey participants ranked workplace safety highly, but 60 percent of them identified workplace stress as the highest safety risk This stress involves multiple aspects, including bullying, threats, assaults, high work volume, and workload. Results about workplace stress showed (1) 64 percent will report workplace bullying; (2) 29 percent have been verbally or physically threatened by a patient or family member in the past year; (3) 10 percent have been assaulted at work by a patient or family member; (4) 53 percent often work through breaks to complete assigned duties; (5) 52 percent often come early or stay late to complete work; (6) 26 percent frequently have a higher workload than they can comfortably handle; and (7) 50 percent feel they should work when sick or injured (ANA Enterprise, 2018, p. 36).

Survey participants identified safe patient handling (26 percent) and mobility and sharps injuries (24 percent) as other areas of safety risks. Most nurses have access to safe patient handling devices, but only 21 percent help select these devices. Safety devices for sharps prevention are common, but only 22 percent are included in their selection. Even with these supports, 57 percent of participants have had musculoskeletal pain at work in the past year and 12 percent have had a sharps injury in the past five years. On-the-job injuries affected 9 percent of participants and 77 percent report these injuries (ANA Enterprise, 2018, pp. 36–37).

Quality of Life

HNHN recommended use of mindfulness, a seven-minute workout, spending time in nature, and self-care. Seventy percent of survey participants rated their health as good or very good and 6 percent rated their health as excellent. Compared to others their age, 10 percent of participants stated their health was excellent and 62 percent rated it as good or very good. While 61 percent believed that access to emotional support is always or often available, 25 percent reported feeling depressed or sad for more than two consecutive weeks (ANA Enterprise, 2018, p. 34).

HNHN's action plan is an easy way to join the initiative and ANA Enterprise has developed multiple resources to support nurses in their journey to health and well-being. There have been notable success stories and this initiative has led the way nationally as a role model for others to follow.

Regional Activities—Improving Provider Work Life (Team Vitality)

The Michigan Health Improvement Alliance (MiHIA) added the Fourth Aim—"improving the work life of healthcare providers, clinicians and staff, known as Provider Well-Being"—to its initiatives in 2016. This addition to the Strategic Business Plan addressed their belief that organizations who care for their staff will have a huge competitive advantage because "happier, healthier providers deliver higher quality care, with better patient satisfaction and are more engaged in their organizations" (MiHIA.org, 2018, p. 5). MiHIA has established a goal: "Establish baseline measurement of and sustainable processes for assessing provider well-being in the region. Repeat assessment annually/periodically to maintain or improve provider well-being" (MiHIA.org, 2018, p. 5). Outcome measurement data is not available at present so this section will address the work of another organization to improve provider work life.

The Vanderbilt University Medical Center Division of Health and Wellness has three highly-developed programs that impact their staff as well as faculty and staff at Vanderbilt University. The Occupational Health Clinic goes beyond basic screening and immunization compliance to provide programs, such as Wellcasts on a variety of topics that may impact all employees. These include heart disease in women, fibroids and their treatment, and stroke prevention and education. Their screening programs are diverse and include noise exposure, animal allergies, and traffic and parking medical screening for employed drivers. This department provides All Aboard weekly where new employees can obtain required health services and learn how to obtain their own health providers and services. The Occupational Health Center staff also provides information about available health and wellness services and regularly visits all facilities and units for easy access by staff (vumc.org, n.d.).

Health Plus's mission is "advancing healthy lifestyle practices" (vumc. org, n.d.). This program offers several options to promote health and well-being. The first is Go for the Gold an incentive program offering up to $240 annually for (1) completing the Compass Health Assessment to identify personal health concerns and ways to improve health; (2) using the Wellness Actions Log to record actions to improve wellness; and (3) watching the Game Plan video which shares tips and practical ideas for health improvement (vumc.org, n.d.). Health Plan also uses Wellness Commodores—staff role models in each department who generate department wellness projects and keep staff informed about the services and programs of Health Plus. Lifestyle Coaching is available free of charge to any employee who wants to improve physical activity, eat healthier, lose weight, stop smoking, or reduce stress. The coach does a face-to-face session to initially check BMI, height, weight, and blood pressure while collaboratively establishing a plan to address strengths, challenges, and goals for improvement. Monthly visits with the coach continue either in-person, via phone, or computer. A follow-up appointment at six months rechecks all measurements and monitors progress (vumc.org, n.d.). For anyone interested in walking as exercise, routes on the Vanderbilt Campus are marked for ease in planning walks of 10- to 40-minute duration (vumc.org, n.d.).

Twice a year, Health Plus offers Control is the Goal for hypertensive staff members to promote healthy choices and blood pressure monitoring. The program has six weekly online modules and recommends blood pressure checks weekly for at least six weeks. If these checks are done by Health Plus staff (Know the Numbers), this information can be used in the Go for the Gold Program. CORE Nutrition is another Health Plus program to learn about healthy foods and offers healthy food samples, practical recipes, and an opportunity to ask questions about healthy nutrition. CORE Nutrition is also available within departments in one- to two-hour time blocks that encourage staff to attend sessions in a relaxed atmosphere (vumc.org, n.d.).

The final Health Plus program is Mindful Break. This unique offering is available in any department that has an empty room with space to accommodate 10 people for up to 20 minutes at a time. The initial session is coordinated by a Health Plus staffer and a department member is trained as leader using Mindful Break materials and observation of the initial session. A recorded meditation and video are available to participants. The leader helps staff members practice breathing and stretching exercises to encourage relaxation (vumc.org, n.d.).

The third program is Work/Life Connections which has the mission "elevating psychological resilience" (vumc.org, n.d.). This program conducts performance coaching for employees, counseling for employees and spouses, and consultation services for leaders addressing performance issues and difficult workplace issues. It also provides programs and resources to enhance faculty and staff resilience. The Resilience Toolkit focuses on attitude, skill set, and lifestyle that encourage employees to handle challenges and stressful events by using multiple options for self-care. Attitude involves being optimistic making social connections, welcoming change, using humor, being grateful, and willing to accept help. Skill Set involves use of mindfulness, communication, problem solving, and emotional intelligence. Lifestyle includes physical activity, good nutrition, and adequate sleep (vumc.org, n.d.).

Beyond traditional EAP services, Vanderbilt's Work/Life Connections also has a Faculty & Physician Wellness Program that provides psychological support to house physicians and spouses as well as the faculty of all eleven Vanderbilt University schools. This program was initiated in 1999 to meet the needs of professionals related to "stress, depression, addiction and other emotional and behavioral issues" (vumc.org, n.d.). Since its inception, over 1,000 physicians and faculty have received care and 95 percent of these were self-referred. Each client works confidentially with both a counselor and a psychiatrist. The program is easy to access and uses a compassionate approach to help clients resolve significant personal and professional issues (vumc.org, n.d.).

The Nurse Wellness Program began in 2002 to provide psychological support to nurses. This specialized service is coordinated by the Work/Life Connections-EAP Nurse Wellness Specialist whose charge is to help nurses focus on self-care so they can care for others. The PostDoc Wellness Program for post-doctoral students is similar to the two discussed above and helps these individuals develop their skills and strengths to establish their professional identities through performance coaching and counseling (vumc.org, n.d.).

These examples illustrate Vanderbilt's commitment to employee health and wellness. The organization has been recognized regionally and nationally for this with numerous awards:

1. One of the Healthiest 100 Workplaces in America in 2014 and 2018 based on sustained successful employee wellness initiatives;
2. Best Employers for Healthy Lifestyles® Award in the Gold category for 2013, 2014, and 2015 for creating changes to support employees' commitment to behavioral changes;
3. Global Healthy Workplace named Vanderbilt second in the world for improving mental and physical health and safety of employees;

4. Healthiest Employers of Middle Tennessee Award 2010–2015 for wellness programs for employees; and

5. 2014 Healthier Tennessee Workplace for the value on health and well-being of staff and faculty [vumc.org, n.d.].

Vanderbilt's three-pronged approach in its wellness and health initiatives is a role model in the region and nationally to improve provider work life and team vitality.

The Future of Provider Work Life (Team Vitality)

Although the Fourth Aim is the most recent addition to the Quadruple Aim, it significantly impacts the success of the other three Aims. National groups like ANA Enterprise and regional employers like Vanderbilt and MiHIA are tackling this Aim to benefit healthcare workers, but more must be done to encourage resilience and mindfulness and eliminate terms like burnout and compassion fatigue. Healthcare teams must learn positive ways to deal with complex stressful work situations and the team members must be ready to support each other beyond just debriefing and use of EAP services. Interprofessional teams who learn together and from each other will be more cohesive. Academic programs must encourage interprofessional education that includes tips and techniques to handle stress in difficult situations. These programs should include a specific course in well-being—physical, personal, emotional, psychological, social, spiritual, and professional—to help participants achieve balance in their lives and work relationships. Lack of work-life balance can result in "depression; lower resilience; job dissatisfaction; and a propensity toward unhealthy lifestyle coping mechanisms" (Hume, 2018, p. 9).

Studies show that these symptoms of poor staff well-being result in increased medical errors and inadequate patient safety. A wellness framework in healthcare organizations provides the foundation for engaging staff members in their health journey. Vanderbilt's model can serve as an example, but each organization in all settings must collaborate with team members to use both a standardized and individual approach to wellness (Hume, 2018).

No one approach works for everyone. Caregivers must realize that without self-care, they can't effectively care for others. Unfortunately, many healthcare personnel don't know how to do this. Leaders, colleagues, other team members, and family can assist individuals in learning how to use self-care activities, such as meditation, relaxation exercises, mindfulness, and supportive relationships. Self-care is a key to resilience or the ability to bounce back from adverse, stressful situations (Kester & Wei, 2018).

This Aim must succeed within the diverse healthcare workforce to improve the health and well-being of providers and the individuals and populations they serve. Education, self-care techniques, and support systems can only work if healthcare team members realize their own needs and take steps to meet them for the benefit of everyone—individual patients/clients, at-risk populations, other team members, and (most of all) themselves.

Nurse Leaders and Improving Provider Work Life (Team Vitality)

Nightingale's Influence

When Florence Nightingale arrived in Scutari, there was chaos in the hospitals there. The Barrack Hospital where she and her nurses worked was overcrowded, unsanitary, and lacking hospital bedding and basic necessities for the wounded. She realized that patient care would be improved if there was teamwork among those providing care. She ensured that her nurses were helpful to physicians and she helped the doctors obtain essential supplies for care delivery. The most overlooked team members were the orderlies who were overworked, underpaid, and poorly fed. They neglected their duties and Nightingale began to train them and recommended benefits for them. Her efforts to improve their health and well-being resulted in improved care and attention by the orderlies to their patients as described by her as "I must pay tribute to the instinctive delicacy, the ready attention of orderlies and patients during all that dreadful period ... the tears come to my eyes as I think how, amidst scenes of loathsome disease and death, there rose above it all the innate dignity, gentleness, and chivalry of the men" (Cook, 1913a, p. 242).

Improving Provider Work Life (Team Vitality)— Nurse Leaders 2020 and Beyond

The nurse leaders profiled in this book shared how they care for themselves so they can care for others. Nurse leaders also play a critical role in helping other team members care for themselves so they can truly care for their patients/clients. They need to build supportive relationships and engagement with team members so they can aid them when stressors arise.

Nurse leaders also need to give meaningful recognition to team members, particularly when the staff member has a challenging or difficult experience at work. This doesn't have to be costly, but it has to be timely. A card of appreciation or a small token can work wonders when someone is experiencing emotional stress. Education, both formal and informal, is another way for nurse leaders to help employees use resilience to deal with stress. Such education helps the individual "identify stressors, be aware of personal triggers, and take part in preferred self-care activities" (Kester &Wei, 2018).

Nurse leaders must also engage staff members in planning interventions to maintain a support network on the unit. Huddles where employees share experiences in a safe, nonthreatening environment can foster a climate of trust and teamwork. The health and well-being of team members must be a priority for leaders and everyone is accountable for success.

15

Preparing Future Nurse Leaders to Address the Quadruple Aim

Future nurse leaders will be responsible for ensuring high quality care to meet the health needs of individuals and at-risk populations using cost effective and efficient approaches within interprofessional team activities. This is not an easy challenge and current orientation for the nurse leader role does not automatically prepare future nurse leaders to address each of these Aims.

The nurse leader role must incorporate ethics, education (both academic and professional development), evidence-based practice, research, diversity, and political savvy and legislative advocacy to successfully address the Quadruple Aim in multiple practice settings.

Ethics

> "Mysticism: to dwell on the unseen, to withdraw ourselves from the things of sense into communion with God—to endeavor to partake of the Divine nature; that is, of Holiness. When we ask ourselves only what is right, or what is the will of God (the same question), then we may truly be said to live in His light."—Florence Nightingale (Cook, 1913b, p. 231)

> The way to live with God is to live with Ideas—not merely to think about ideals, but to do and suffer for them. Those who have to work on men and women must above all things, have their Spiritual Ideal, their purpose, ever present. The "mystical" state is the essence of common sense.—Cook, 1913b, p. 235

Florence Nightingale was a mystic who believed that caring for individuals required a spiritual focus and working for the good of others. Although she did not define this as ethical practice, her clinical performance demonstrated ethical behavior throughout her career. She also ensured that her protégées and students in the Nightingale School adhered to ethical standards in caring for patients.

Nurse leaders today serve as role models for ethical practice and this knowledge must be shared with future nurse leaders as they ensure that individuals and at-risk populations receive ethical care.

The first Code of Ethics for Nurses with Interpretive Statements originated in the late 1800s as the American Nurses Association (ANA) was founded. This Code evolved over many years and continues to do so today. It was first adopted by the American Nurses Association in 1950 as the first professional ethics code. Today, it serves as a guide for all practicing nurses and has three purposes: (1) a concise statement of individual and aggregate nurses' "ethical values, obligations, duties, and professional ideals"; (2) the ethical standard for the nursing profession; and (3) a representation of nursing's perception of its obligation to society (ANA, 2015, Preface viii).

The ANA Code of Ethics with Interpretive Statements is dynamic and continues to change as society and the social determinants of health change in the United States and globally. It is applicable to all nurses in all settings and future nurse leaders must understand and adhere to its provisions and interpretive statements in their practice. The provisions are broad statements about nurses' duties and responsibilities. The interpretive statements provide specific information about how to apply each provision to current nursing practice. While provisions do not change significantly over time, interpretive statements change at least each decade as nursing practice and the social context of care evolve (ANA, 2015).

The terminology reflects recognized language that is inclusive and can be easily understood. For example, the Code uses the word "patient" throughout the narrative. Although nurses also care for "clients," the term "patient" refers to "clients or consumers of healthcare as well as to individuals or groups" (ANA, 2015, Introduction xi). Ethics and morality are distinguished from each other in the Code and morality focuses on "personal values, character, or conduct of individuals or groups within communities" (ANA, 2015, Introduction xi). Ethics formally studies that morality from numerous perspectives as "a branch of philosophy or theology in which one reflects on morality" (ANA, 2015, Introduction xi-xii). It addresses morality issues and questions in behavior. The Code of Ethics for Nurses with Interpretive Statements includes a glossary of terms for the first time in the 2015 edition. ANA's Ethics webpage contains links to the Code and the Introduction is a new feature that provides information about the structure and terminology of the Code. The Steering Committee for the Revision of the Code of Ethics for Nurses with Interpretive Statements simplified and clarified the content to make it easier to use in the current complex healthcare environment (ANA, 2015).

The Code has nine provisions that focus on three aspects of nurses' performance. The first three provisions address nurses' commitments and fundamental values. The second three provisions address nurses' loyalty and duty and the final three provisions address nurses' duties and responsibilities beyond interactions with individual patients. The interpretive statements provide specific guidance for nurses in practice (ANA, 2015).

Future nurse leaders must be conversant and knowledgeable about all nine provisions of the Code of Ethics for Nurses with Interpretive Statements if they are to address all Quadruple Aim measures in their practice settings. Each provision impacts at least one measure in the Quadruple Aim Framework. **Provision 1** "The nurse practices with compassion and respect for the inherent dignity, worth, and unique attributes of every person" (ANA, 2015, p. 1). Nurse leaders' adherence to this provision enables them to treat people with dignity and develop relationships with individuals that will improve their experience of care (Quadruple Aim Goal 1). A climate of trust and acceptance will enable nurse leaders and their colleagues to respect patient (individual) decisions about care. If these decisions are detrimental to the person's health, the nurse leaders must address choices that will help the individual modify behavior and reduce risks. Social determinants of health (Quadruple Aim Goal 3) are affected by this provision as nurse leaders focus on factors that influence a person's health status. This includes advocating for appropriate interventions and leading improvement in community structures that may adversely impact individual and population health (Quadruple Aim Goal 2). Nurse leaders also recognize that individuals must be included and supported in decision-making about their care. This is particularly important in end of life decisions where the individual's decisions about life support, resuscitation, nutrition, and hydration require the nurse leader to ensure compassionate care in accordance with the individual's needs (Quadruple Aim Goal 1). This provision also addresses the nurse leader's relationships with others, including colleagues. Treating others with dignity and respect fosters collaboration and team vitality (Quadruple Aim Goal 4).

Provision 2 "The nurse's primary commitment is to the patient, whether an individual, family group, community, or population" (ANA, 2015, p. 5). Nurse leaders must be committed to the individual's or population's health and well-being and ensure that the plan of care is individualized with input from the individual and significant other(s). Care planning and implementation require candid discussions to enhance decision-making by the individual or member of the population (Quadruple Aim Goal 1 and Quadruple Aim Goal 2). Nurse leaders may experience conflicts of interest in this provision based on their budgetary responsibilities. Their organizations' delivery systems may be impacted by healthcare financing issues that may conflict with the interests of individuals or members of high-risk populations. When this is the case, the nurse leader should withdraw from participating in this particular situation (Quadruple Aim Goal 3). The nurse leader must collaborate with other healthcare team members "to provide safe, high-quality, patient-centered healthcare" (ANA, 2015, p. 6). The nurse leader's primary commitment to the patient, whether an individual or a member of a high-risk population, requires ensuring that everyone relevant to the patient's health and well-being is involved the care delivery and decision-making process (Quadruple Aim Goal 4). The nurse leader also maintains professional boundaries when working with individuals, members of populations, and colleagues and avoids inappropriate personal relationships to focus on commitment to the individual or population member and that person's health needs (Quadruple Aim Goal 1 and Quadruple Aim Goal 2).

Provision 3 "The nurse promotes, advocates for, and protects the rights, health, and safety of the patient" (ANA, 2015, p. 9). The nurse leader must protect the privacy and confidentiality of information and communication with individuals or population members. Adherence to policies and procedures that protect clinical and personal information is essential and nurse leaders must ensure that there is no disclosure of any personal information to protect patient rights (Quadruple Aim Goal 1 and Quadruple Aim Goal 2). The nurse leader's role in protecting participants in research studies assures informed consent and addresses concerns about vulnerable groups such as "children, cognitively impaired persons, economically or educational disadvantaged persons, fetuses, older adults, pregnant women, prisoners, and underserved populations" (ANA, 2015, pp. 10–11). Nurse leaders' advocacy extends to monitoring and reporting deviations from acceptable research protocols (Quadruple Aim Goal 1; Quadruple Aim Goal 2; Quadruple Aim Goal 3). Nurse leaders promote a culture of safety by investigating near misses or errors with a focus on correction or remediation to prevent future recurrence. They are responsible for ensuring that nurses are competent to deliver care that safeguards patient safety and promotes positive care outcomes. They also must protect patient health and safety by addressing and reporting inappropriate, questionable, or impaired practice (Quadruple Aim Goal 1 and Quadruple Aim Goal 2).

Provision 4 "The nurse has authority, accountability, and responsibility for nursing practice; makes decisions; and takes action consistent with the obligation to promote health and to provide optimal care" (ANA, 2015, p. 15). Nurse leaders understand that the scope of nursing practice continues to change and evolve. Each nurse is responsible for the care delivered to individuals and members of at-risk populations in his/her charge as well as demonstrating accountability for his/her own practice (Quadruple Aim Goal 1 and Quadruple Aim Goal 2). Nursing practice is diverse and "includes independent direct nursing care activities; care as ordered by an authorized healthcare provider; care coordination; evaluation of interventions; delegation of nursing interventions; and other responsibilities such as teaching, research, and administration" (ANA, 2015, p. 15). Nurse leaders also demonstrate responsibility for patient care by ensuring that nurses reporting to them are competent and have access to appropriate resources when caring for patients. They safeguard others through standards of professional practice, peer review, quality improvement initiatives, and research projects. Nurse leaders also include nurses in organization committees that address ethics, patient safety, and quality of care so they can participate in the decision-making team (Quadruple Aim Goal 1; Quadruple Aim Goal 2; Quadruple Aim Goal 4). Nurse leaders create open dialogue with healthcare personnel to ensure appropriate assignments and delegation of tasks (Quadruple Aim Goal 4).

Provision 5 "The nurse owes the same duties to self as to others, including the responsibility to promote health and safety, preserve wholeness of character and integrity, maintain competence, and continue personal and professional growth" (ANA, 2015, p. 19). Nurse leaders realize that they owe themselves the same duties they accord to others. Their personal safety, health, and well-being help them improve their professional and personal life by balancing work and personal responsibilities (Quadruple Aim Goal 4). To achieve this balance, nurse leaders "should eat a healthy diet, exercise, get sufficient rest, maintain family and personal relationships, engage in adequate leisure and recreational activities, and attend to spiritual or religious needs" (ANA. 2015, p. 19). Nurse leaders integrate both personal and professional values to express ideas that are central to situations. They are careful to avoid undue influence when individuals are making informed decisions about their care and are respectful of others' beliefs (Quadruple Aim Goal 1 and Quadruple Aim Goal 2). Nurse leaders also preserve the integrity of nurses by responding promptly to concerns about moral distress threats, and abuse by others—patients, families, colleagues. Their intervention must protect the nurse while providing for patient safety (Quadruple Aim Goal 4). Nurse leaders must demonstrate a commitment to lifelong learning to achieve professional growth and routinely self-evaluate their performance to maintain competence. They also must continue personal growth with a variety of activities that enhance their knowledge and self-awareness and enable them to improve their work life as a result (Quadruple Aim Goal 4).

Provision 6 "The nurse, through individual and collective effort, establishes, maintains, and improves the ethical environment of the work setting and conditions of employment that are conducive to safe, quality healthcare" (ANA, 2015, p. 23). Nurse leaders ensure that the work environment supports nurses to use these virtues in their daily practice—"knowledge, skill, wisdom, patience, compassion, honesty, altruism, and courage" (ANA, 2015, p. 23). These virtues promote caring, respect, and communication between all colleagues that benefits the healthcare team and the individuals they serve (Quadruple Aim Goal 1 and Quadruple Aim Goal 4). Policies and procedures can establish expectations for ethical professional practice and peer pressure can positively impact performance expectation within the work group (Quadruple Aim Goal 4). Other factors can positively or negatively affect the practice environment including "compensation systems, disciplinary procedures, ethics committees and consulting services, grievance mechanisms that prevent reprisal, health and safety initiatives, organizational processes and structures, performance standards, policies addressing discrimination and incivility, position descriptions" (ANA, 2015, p. 24). Nurse leaders have responsibility for influencing the healthcare environment to promote mutual support and respectful communication within the healthcare team (Quadruple Aim Goal 4). They also are responsible for addressing concerns within organizational channels to initiate positive change. They should never tolerate a work environment that is morally unacceptable and can seek support from professional organizations to ensure safe practice environments for nurses, patients, and other healthcare professionals (ANA, 2015, p. 25).

Provision 7 "The nurse, in all roles and settings, advances the profession through research and scholarly inquiry, professional standards development, and the generation of both nursing and health policy" (ANA, 2015, p. 27). Nurse leaders advance the nursing profession by engaging in scholarly inquiry that expands the discipline's body of knowledge. They ensure that research is conducted ethically and that the rights of research subjects are protected (Quadruple Aim Goal 1 and Quadruple Aim Goal 2). Dissemination of results is essential for knowledge development and can result in educational and clinical innovation and interprofessional collaboration (Quadruple Aim Goal 4). Nurse leaders enable nurses to practice according to professional practice standards that ensure quality patient care (Quadruple Aim Goal 1 and Quadruple Aim Goal 2). Nurse leaders also serve as leaders and mentors on organization or agency policy committees and participate in activities about healthcare locally, regionally, nationally, or globally to advocate for health policy development (Quadruple Aim Goal 3).

Provision 8 "The nurse collaborates with other health professionals and the public to protect human rights, promote health diplomacy, and reduce health disparities" (ANA, 2015, p. 31). Nurse leaders believe "that health is a universal human right" (ANA, 2015, p. 31). This right has implications that are "economic, political, social and cultural" (ANA, 2015, p. 31). For individuals and population members to achieve the best possible health and well-being requires multiple resources that develop their utmost potential (Quadruple Aim Goal 1 and Quadruple Aim Goal 2). These resources include "access to healthcare, emergency care, and trauma care; basic sanitation; education concerning the prevention, treatment, and control of prevailing health problems; food security; immunizations; injury prevention; prevention and control of locally endemic diseases and vectors; public education concerning health promotion and maintenance; potable water; and reproductive healthcare" (ANA, 2015, p. 31). Nurse leaders must address social determinants of health to help individuals and population groups decrease health disparities and reduce per capita healthcare costs (Quadruple Aim Goal 3). This requires collaboration with multiple individuals, groups, and community organizations to educate the public and address health barriers (Quadruple Aim Goal 4). These barriers include "poverty, homelessness, unsafe living conditions, abuse and violence, and lack of access" (ANA, 2015, p. 32). Nurse leaders must be sensitive to cultural diversity in addressing these issues. When human rights are jeopardized, they must respond through collaboration with public health officials and other healthcare team members to protect the public (Quadruple Aim Goal 4).

Provision 9 "The profession of nursing, collectively through its professional organizations, must articulate nursing values, maintain the integrity of the profession, and integrate principles of social justice into nursing and health policy" (ANA, 2015, p. 35). Nurse leaders realize that their professional organizations and associations communicate nursing values to the public as their representatives. If these organizations present a unified message, they can positively influence health globally and social justice (ANA, 2015). The Code of Ethics for Nurses with Interpretive Statements is a contract between the profession and society that defines nurses' ethical responsibility to patients, colleagues, other health professionals, and society. Nursing organizations and nurse leaders advocate for change that improves the health of individuals, members of at-risk populations, and healthcare locally, regionally, nationally, and globally (Quadruple Aim 1 and Quadruple Aim 2). Nurse leaders must address social determinants of health with legislators as well as agencies and organizations that are involved in health issues. They must also join with their professional organizations to address regulatory and legislative topics that impact the nursing profession and the health of the public, such as the impact of environmental issues on health that adversely affects the health of poor individuals with escalating costs (Quadruple Aim Goal 1; Quadruple Aim Goal 2; Quadruple Aim Goal 3; Quadruple Aim Goal 4).

The Nightingale Pledge

This nursing narrative about ethics would be incomplete without including the Nightingale pledge which was written by a committee chaired by Lystra Gretter, a nursing instructor at the Farrand Training School for Nurses in Detroit, Michigan. It is an adaptation of the physicians' Hippocratic Oath and was first used by the Farrand graduating class of 1893. While the Pledge represents ethical conduct for nurses and continues to be used in nursing graduation ceremonies, it has been adapted over the years and is not without controversy. The original Pledge which is shown here has been revised to address reference to God based on nurses' diverse religious observances. Other changes reflect collaboration, rather than loyalty to the physician and language about living a life of purity may be interpreted differently today than in 1893 (Miracle, 2009, pp. 145–146). Nevertheless, the Pledge is applicable to ethical performance and meaningful in relation to the Quadruple Aim measures:

> "I solemnly pledge myself before God and in the presence of this assembly:
> To pass my life in purity and to practice my profession faithfully.
> I will abstain from whatever is deleterious and mischievous, and will not take or knowingly administer any harmful drug.
> I will do all in my power to maintain and elevate the standard of my profession, and will hold in confidence all personal matters committed to my keeping and all family affairs coming to my knowledge in this practice of my profession.
> With loyalty will I endeavor to aid the physician in his work, and devote myself to the welfare of those committed to my care" [Miracle, 2009, p. 145].

Academic Education

> The Committee of her [Nightingale's] Council met the Governors of the [St. Thomas] Hospital, and an agreement was arrived at for the foundation of the Nightingale School. The basis of the agreement was that the Hospital

was to provide facilities for the training, and the Nightingale Fund to pay the cost, including the payment of the
nurses themselves. In May 1860, advertisements were
inserted in the public press inviting candidates for admission, and on June 24 fifteen probationers were admitted
for a year's training. Thus on a modest scale, but with
a vast amount of forethought, was launched the scheme
which was destined to found the modern art and practice
of nursing.—Cook, 1913a, p. 459

For a long time, the Nightingale model of service in exchange for education
was the only way to become an educated nurse. Today, there continue to
be diverse avenues to academic nursing education. Licensed Practical or
Licensed Vocational Nurses (LPNs/LVNs) receive 12 months of technical
education at a community college or technical school. Upon successful
program completion, graduates are eligible to take a licensing examination.
Upon passage, they can provide direct nursing care to the limits of their
training and licensure under the direction of physicians and registered
nurses (BLS.gov, n.d.).

Education for registered nurses began in the United States when Diploma schools affiliated with hospitals began as one-year programs with
room and board in exchange for providing patient care services to the facility. Over the years, these programs became three years in length, but service continued to be emphasized with little attention to liberal arts courses.
Today few of these schools remain, but their students now receive education
in arts and sciences in collaboration with local colleges or universities and
are no longer used as supplemental staffing for the affiliated hospital. Upon
program completion, graduates must successfully pass a licensing examination to practice as an entry-level registered nurse (NursingSchoolPrograms.
com, n.d.).

The Associate of Science in Nursing (ASN/ADN) is a two-year education program for nursing students conducted in community colleges. This
option was popular in the past because it meets all requirements to pursue
bachelor's and advanced degrees. For many people, it was a less expensive
option than a four-year bachelor of science in nursing (BSN) degree and
enabled graduates to pursue the BSN while working and earning a living.
Today, many schools are affiliated with colleges offering BSNs and nurses
who have successfully passed the licensing examination (NCLEX) can use
accelerated programs to attain the BSN. Many employers also offer tuition
reimbursement to help defray the cost of the BSN degree (NursingSchool.
org, n.d.).

Today the bachelor of science in nursing (BSN) degree is the preferred entry level for registered nurses. As previously stated, the Institute of Medicine (IOM) in its report *The Future of Nursing: Leading Change, Advancing Health* focused on the importance of nursing education in its "Recommendation 4: Increase the proportion of nurses with a baccalaureate degree to 80 percent by 2020" (IOM, 2011, p. 12). Academic nurse leaders were charged with collaborating "to increase the proportion of nurses with a baccalaureate degree from 50 to 80 percent by 2020." While this goal has not yet been achieved, the American Association of Colleges of Nursing (AACN) commissioned a study in 2015 to determine how academic nursing can advance its effect on this recommendation and healthcare transformation at all levels (Enders, Morin & Pawlak, 2016).

Nursing academic education plays an indelible role in the ability of registered nurse leaders to fully address the Quadruple Aim Framework in their practice and includes another recommendation from the Institute of Medicine in its report: "Prepare and enable nurses to lead change to advance health" (IOM, 2011, p. 14). This recommendation requires academic educators to prepare nurse leaders for future roles in transforming healthcare.

The AACN project titled *Advancing Healthcare Transformation: A New Era for Academic Nursing* was a comprehensive study to identify the impact of academic nursing on Academic Health Centers (AHCs) where many nursing academic programs are currently affiliated. Interviews were also conducted with stakeholders in both AHC and non–ACH healthcare organizations to determine issues and opportunities for academic nursing (Enders, Morin & Pawlak, 2016).

Academic health centers and non-academic healthcare organizations face the challenges of "changing economics, market consolidation, generational changes in the healthcare workforce, and an increasing focus on chronic disease prevention and management" (Enders, Morin & Pawlak, 2016, p. 2). They must streamline processes by delivering care more efficiently and effectively and nurses are integral in this process change as advocates for individuals and at-risk populations (Quadruple Aim 1; Quadruple Aim 2; Quadruple Aim 3). The report's findings about the current alignment between academic nursing and academic health centers revealed obstacles that must be overcome. Here are the findings.

1. Academic nursing cannot function as a full partner in the transformation of healthcare due to organizational limitations.
2. Academic health center leaders are aware of the lack of opportunity for partnership with academic nursing and are willing to try new approaches.
3. Lack of funding for academic nursing is a barrier to enhancing its

role in institutional leadership and healthcare transformation [Enders, Morin & Pawlak, 2016, p. 2].

Clinical innovation is essential for academic and non-academic health organizations to meet the needs of individuals and populations cost effectively and efficiently. Nursing academic faculty can facilitate clinical innovations if they become more involved in clinical practice in partnership with organization leaders. They can promote nursing research that is patient and community focused, but they must be at the table for this to happen (Quadruple Aim 1; Quadruple Aim 2; Quadruple Aim 3).

The report made six recommendations for organization leaders to facilitate this academic-organization partnership.

1. The first recommendation asked organizations to adopt a new vision for academic nursing: "Academic nursing is a full partner in healthcare delivery, education, and research that is integrated and funded across all professions and missions in the Academic Health System" (Enders, Morin & Pawlak, 2016, p. 3). This vision includes these elements:
   a. participation by academic nursing in governance within the health system;
   b. increased leadership in care delivery and clinical practice by academic faculty (Quadruple Aim 1);
   c. partnership within the healthcare system and its professionals to evolve and grow nursing research programs with academic faculty (Quadruple Aim 1 and Quadruple Aim 2);
   d. partnership between academic faculty and the organization to develop training programs and collaborative plans for the workforce (Quadruple Aim 4);
   e. assimilation of academic faculty in initiatives to improve population health (Quadruple Aim 2); and
   f. commitment for leadership development of future nurse leaders [Quadruple Aim 4].

2. Initiatives should encourage academic faculty to be involved in clinical practice and align the organization's clinical service to the school's mission (Quadruple Aim 1).

3. The school of nursing and the academic health system must partner to prepare future nurses at multiple education levels to meet the system's clinical requirements, including nursing leadership development courses (Quadruple Aim 1 and Quadruple Aim 4).

4. Academic faculty must partner with clinicians and organization leaders to implement accountable care programs (Quadruple Aim 3).

5. Nursing research activities should be coordinated to integrate the work of academic and clinical nurse researchers into practice that benefits both the organization and the community (Quadruple Aim 2).

6. AACN and organization leaders must develop an agenda that aligns with the Quadruple Aim by advocating "growth in NIH budget to support nursing-led research; increased funding support for the training of nurse-scientists; expansion of the Graduate Nurse Education (GNE) Demonstration; heightened advocacy for scope of practice changes to enable nurses to take on the clinical roles they are trained to perform; and support for academic nursing leadership in clinical care delivery" (Enders, Morin & Pawlak, 2016, p. 4).

Academic education prepares nurses to provide care in multiple settings such as hospitals, medical offices, outpatient clinics, home care agencies, and hospice/palliative care sites. New education models are required for future nurses to deliver care for population health (Quadruple Aim 2). Curriculum changes also include interprofessional education, where multiple disciplines learn from and with each other (Quadruple Aim 4). Academic faculty must provide education that prepares their graduates to function in outpatient settings to address healthcare organizations' focus on lower cost locations (Quadruple Aim 3). Academic nursing plays a significant role in research "on population health, chronic disease management models, and collaborative care approaches translated into new care models that improve the health of patients and the population" (Enders, Morin & Pawlak, 2016, p. 7). This research addresses Quadruple Aim 2 and Quadruple Aim 4.

Despite the value of academic nursing education in healthcare, academic nurse leaders have not been integrated with health systems and academic medicine in decision-making. This lack of alignment is a barrier to professional collaboration. Value-based care results in a move from specialty services by healthcare organizations to a focus on population health (Quadruple Aim 2 and Quadruple Aim 3). Academic nurse leaders have the ability to educate nurses in the essential elements of caring for at-risk populations. For this to benefit these individuals and the health system, an alliance is necessary between academic nurse leaders, the health system, and other professionals in an interprofessional environment (Enders, Morin & Pawlak, 2016).

The report offered strategies to ally academic nursing with health systems. These strategies include

1. creation of clinical leadership roles for nursing faculty and appointing organization nurse leaders to faculty roles. This integration will require financing models to achieve education benefits for

organization nurses and clinical innovations that reduce costs (Quadruple Aim 3);

   2. partnership between academic faculty and clinical nurse leaders to redesign service delivery models that emphasize population health and ambulatory care (Quadruple Aim 2);

   3. inclusion of academic nursing in clinical practice that generates income for the school of nursing;

   4. expansion of joint appointments to facilitate team-based clinical practice (Quadruple Aim 4);

   5. promotion of nurse-managed clinics to meet the needs of at-risk populations (Quadruple Aim 2); and

   6. use of contractual arrangements between the health system and the school to improve clinical and financial results [Enders, Morin & Pawlak, 2016].

Academic nursing education can play a significant role in transforming healthcare by partnering with academic health centers, healthcare organizations, and other professionals to advance population health and community-centered care. Barriers must be overcome and an incremental approach may be valuable. If nurse leaders are going to address the Quadruple Aim Framework, academic education must provide essential tools for them to succeed.

Nursing Professional Development

> "A woman who thinks in herself: 'Now I am a full Nurse, a skilled Nurse, I have learnt all that there is to be learnt'— take my word for it, she does not know what a Nurse is, and she never will know; she is gone back already."—Florence Nightingale (Cook, 1913b, p. 264)

   Florence Nightingale knew the importance of lifelong learning and shared that with her probationers at the Nightingale School. It is equally important for today's practicing nurses.

   Although excellent academic education is vital in preparing nurse graduates for entry to practice, continuing professional development is essential for nurses, especially nurse leaders, to advance in the profession and initiate changes that address the Quadruple Aim Framework. There are numerous approaches that encourage lifelong learning, including conferences, symposia, online continuing education courses, self-studies, workshops, simulation, and virtual learning activities.

In this context, the American Nurses Association has established education as a standard of professional performance for practicing nurses. Standard 12 states, "The registered nurse seeks knowledge and competence that reflects current nursing practice and promotes futuristic thinking" (American Nurses Association, 2015, p. 76). Such standards depict competent performance by nurses that demonstrate accountability "for their professional actions to themselves, their healthcare consumers, their peers, and ultimately to society" (American Nurses Association, 2015, p. 5). Lifelong learning enables nurse leaders to support individuals, at-risk populations, and other members of the interprofessional team in accordance with the Quadruple Aim Framework. For many nurses, this encompasses national specialty certification in addition to competency validation. Competencies related to this standard demonstrate compliance and are dependent on the circumstances of the nurse's role. Viewing the Education standard from the Quadruple Aim Framework, let's see how the recommended competencies enable nurse leaders to address the Quadruple aim measures.

1. Identification of learning needs based on roles and nursing knowledge (ANA, 2015, p. 76) enables the nurse to critically assess his/her current knowledge base about all four Quadruple Aim measures and determine which measures will require additional education. For example, the nurse leader may be very knowledgeable about the nurse's role in individual perception of care (Quadruple aim 1) and caring for at-risk populations (Quadruple Aim 20), but needs additional education about fiscal management to reduce per capita cost of care (Quadruple Aim 3) and how to promote team vitality (Quadruple Aim 4).

2. Participation in learning activities on an ongoing basis about nursing, interprofessional knowledge, and specialized topics (ANA, 2015, p. 76) will enable the nurse to address the above learning needs as well as the importance of interprofessional education in improving provider work life (team vitality).

3. Registered nurses must mentor nurses who are new to their roles to support, orient, and enculturate them into the practice environment (ANA, 2015, p. 76). This is a vital competency for nurse leaders to ensure that new nurses can practice in accordance with the Quadruple Aim Framework. They must learn to provide safe, quality, cost effective care to individuals and populations as contributing members of interprofessional teams.

4. Nurses must be committed to lifelong learning by self-reflection and analysis for personal and professional growth (ANA, 2015, p. 76).

This reflects the first two competencies—identification of learning needs and participation in learning activities on an ongoing basis.

5. Nurses must pursue experiences reflecting current practice "to maintain and advance knowledge, skills, abilities, attitudes, and judgment in clinical practice or role performance" (ANA, 2015, p. 76). It is important for nurse leaders to seek opportunities that enhance their performance in addressing all four Quadruple Aim measures in the context of their professional role.

6. Nurses must attain "knowledge and skills relative to the role, population, specialty, setting, and global or local health situation" (ANA, 2015, p. 76). Nurse leaders do not practice in a vacuum. Meeting the needs of individuals and populations for high quality, cost effective care requires ongoing learning and application in practice by nurse leaders (Quadruple Aim 1; Quadruple Aim 2; Quadruple Aim 3). Since nurse leaders also play an integral role in promoting provider work life on interprofessional teams, this competency enables them to use their knowledge and skills to support team growth (Quadruple Aim 4).

7. Nurses must engage in informal and formal dialogue "to address issues in nursing practice as an application of education and knowledge" (ANA, 2015, p. 76). Nurse leaders interact with multiple stakeholders as they address the Quadruple Aim Framework. They bring expertise acquired from education and their clinical knowledge to share expert knowledge about efficient, cost-effective care delivery for individuals and at-risk populations (Quadruple Aim 1; Quadruple Ain 2; Quadruple Aim 3).

8. Nurses must adapt patient/family education to meet their needs for information (ANA, 2015, p. 76). Nurse leaders must ensure that each nurse providing patient/family education is knowledgeable and able to modify education to meet the unique learning needs of individuals and their family members or significant others (Quadruple Aim 1).

9. Nurses must share "educational findings, experiences, and ideas with peers" (ANA, 2015, p. 76). Nurse leaders' pursuit of lifelong learning provides them with valuable data and their experiences with the Quadruple Aim measures enables them create dialogue that will benefit both individuals and at-risk populations (Quadruple Aim 1 and Quadruple Aim 2).

10. Nurses must help other nurses adjust to new roles through "role modeling, encouraging, and sharing pertinent information relative to optimal care delivery" (ANA, 2015, p. 76). Helping other nurses succeed is a paramount responsibility of nurse leaders. They have respon-

sibility and accountability for the care that individuals receive in their work setting. Their support and interaction are essential to ensuring that nurses in new roles succeed for the benefit of the individuals they care for and themselves. These new nurses must be welcomed into the healthcare team and learn to provide optimal care delivery for the team to fully function in delivering care by collaborating with the individual patient at the center of care (Quadruple Aim 1 and Quadruple Aim 4).

11. Nurses must promote "a work environment supportive of ongoing education of healthcare professionals" (ANA, 2015, p. 76). Nurse leaders are accountable for the work environment of their unit(s) in the employment setting. They must demonstrate by their actions that ongoing learning by the healthcare team is essential to truly meet the needs of individuals (patients) and members of at-risk populations (Quadruple Aim 1 and Quadruple Aim 2). Nurse leaders' support of interprofessional education also develops the healthcare team's ability to work together and support each other (Quadruple Aim 4).

12. Nurses must compile "a professional portfolio that provides evidence of individual competence and lifelong learning" (ANA, 2015, p. 76). Nurse leaders also have the responsibility to continue their learning and document it to validate their commitment to the profession and those it serves.

Another national nursing organization, the Association for Nursing Professional Development (ANPD), defines nursing professional development practice by establishing its own standards of practice and standards of professional performance for this nursing specialty. Its standard on education is specific to the nursing professional development (NPD) practitioner: "The nursing professional development practitioner maintains current knowledge and competency in nursing and professional development practice" (ANPD, 2016, p. 44). NPD practitioners engage in environmental scanning for changes in standards of care, practice problems or opportunities for improvement that denote learning needs and analyze data to determine practice gaps. For example, if nurse leaders are addressing lack of team vitality of nurses in interprofessional teams (Quadruple Aim 4), the NPD practitioner can identify learning needs and use data to validate the practice opportunity. After identifying desired outcomes, the NPD practitioner develops a plan to achieve the desired results and implements the plan in coordination with other stakeholders to ensure a positive learning environment. Then, the NPD practitioner evaluates progress toward outcome attainment—enhanced team vitality by nurses. To fulfill these standards of practice—assessment of practice gaps; identification of learning needs; outcomes identification; planning; implementation (coordination, facilitation of positive learning and practice environments, consultation); and evaluation (ANPD, 2016, p. 15)—the NPD practitioner must meet the ANPD standard of professional performance for Education (ANPD, 2016).

Evidence-Based Practice

> Miss Nightingale's proposed forms "would enable the mortality in hospitals, and also the mortality from particular diseases, injuries, and operations, to be ascertained with accuracy; and these facts, together with the duration of cases, would enable the value of particular methods of treatment and of special operations to be brought to statistical proof. The sanitary state of the hospital itself could likewise be ascertained"—Cook, 1913a, p. 430

In an era where standards were inadequate, Nightingale's emphasis on statistical analysis was an opportunity to seek evidence to improve healthcare practices. Nurse leaders voice their support for implementing evidence-based nursing practice in their organizations. They realize that evidence-based care "improves healthcare quality and safety as well as patient outcomes, and it reduces costs and enhances nurses' professional satisfaction" (Valimaki, Partanen & Haggman-Laitila, 2018, p. 424). Use of evidence has the potential to achieve all four Quadruple Aim measures in practice and nurse leaders must make evidence-based practice a priority for themselves and the healthcare team to fully address the Quadruple Aim Framework.

Evidence-based practice is often not a top budget priority although quality and safety are nurse leaders' major priorities. Achieving success in quality and safety requires attention to evidence-based care. Nurse leaders must incorporate evidence-based practice if they want to improve quality and safety and they belong together.

What are the barriers to using evidence-based practice by nurses in the United States?

1. Nurses lack time to read and implement evidence in practice;
2. nurses do not have authority to change procedures for patient care;
3. nurses do not have support from healthcare team members to use evidence-based nursing practice; and

4. nurse leaders and managers are resistant to using evidence-based practice [Valimaki, Partanen & Haggman-Laitila, 2018, p. 424].

Since evidence-based practice by nurses is integral to attaining the Quadruple Aim measures, these barriers must be overcome, especially resistance by nurse leaders who should be spearheading this initiative. Nurse leaders must be knowledgeable about the seven-step evidence-based practice (EBP) process. Each step builds on the previous step.

1. Step 0: Develop an evidence-based environment and culture that nurtures a "spirit of inquiry" (Beckett & Melnyk, 2018, p. 412);
2. Step 1: Ask a PICO(T) question
   a. P=Population to be studied and their characteristics;
   b. I=Intervention or area of interest;
   c. C=Comparison intervention or group;
   d. O=Outcome to be achieved;
   e. T=Time to achieve the outcome (if relevant to study) (Beckett & Melnyk, 2018, p. 412);
3. Step 2: Seek the best available evidence;
4. Step 3: Critically evaluate the evidence;
5. Step 4: Make the best clinical decision by incorporating clinical expertise and patient preferences with the evidence;
6. Step 5: Evaluate outcome(s) of the evidence-based practice change; and
7. Step 6: Disseminate the results of the change [Beckett & Melnyk, 2018, p. 412].

Nurse leaders must demonstrate competence in using all steps of the EBP process so they can help their colleagues understand and use evidence in practice. Luckily, there are competencies for nurses that can help them and their facilities achieve "high-value healthcare, including enhancing the quality and reliability of healthcare, improving health outcomes, and reducing variations in care and costs" (Melnyk, Gallagher-Ford, Long, & Fineout-Overholt, 2014, p. 5). Until recently, there was no certification available in evidence-based practice (EBP). The America Board of Specialty Nursing Certification now offers "the first interprofessional certificate of added qualification (CAQ) in EBP" (Beckett & Melnyk, 2018, p. 413). The written examination is based on 24 evidence-based practice competencies and health professionals who demonstrate EBP competence and have "completed an EBP change proposal, or developed an EBP implementation project, can apply for the CAQ in EBP" (Beckett & Melnyk, 2018, p. 413). To sit for the 50-question examination, the applicant must demonstrate evidence of a graduate level EBP course or completion of "an intense 5-day EBP immersion" (Beckett & Melnyk, 2018, p. 413). This credential can validate the nurse leader's skills in evidence-based practice to self, other healthcare professionals, and the organization.

What are these competencies? Several reflect the seven-step EBP process previously discussed and others reflect advanced practice nursing. The competencies for practicing registered nurses include

a. seeking to improve the quality of care by questioning current clinical practices;

b. reviewing data within the organization—e.g., quality improvement data, safety reports, patient assessment data, patient outcomes data—to describe clinical issues or problems with internal evidence;

c. participating in developing PICO(T) clinical questions;

d. searching for research data to find answers to clinically focused questions;

e. critically appraising evidence such as evidence-based procedures and policies, and clinical practice guidelines;

f. participating in critically rating published research study results for their "strength and applicability to practice" (Melnyk, Gallagher-Ford, Long, & Fineout-Overholt, 2014, p. 11);

g. determining strength and applicability to clinical practice of a body of evidence through evaluation and synthesis;

h. systematically gathering practice data (e.g., quality outcomes data, patient assessment data, patient safety data) "as internal evidence for clinical decision-making in the care of individuals, groups, and populations" (Melnyk, Gallagher-Ford, Long, & Fineout-Overholt, 2014, p. 11);

i. planning evidence-based clinical practice changes by incorporating internal and external evidence;

j. implementing practice changes to improve care delivery processes and patient outcomes by integrating clinical expertise, evidence, and patient preferences;

k. evaluating the outcomes of evidence-based practice decisions to determine best practices for individuals, groups, and populations;

l. disseminating best practices based on evidence that "improve quality of care and patient outcomes" (Melnyk, Gallagher-Ford, Long, & Fineout-Overholt, 2014, p. 11); and

m. sustaining a practice culture that is evidence-based through organizational and individual strategies [Melnyk, Gallagher-Ford, Long, & Fineout-Overholt, 2014].

The above EBP competencies are applicable to all practicing registered nurses. In addition to these competencies, advanced practice nurses and nurse leaders should attain the following competencies to lead evidence-based practice in healthcare:

1. conduct an exhaustive search of research generated evidence on the clinical practice issue or problem;
2. critically evaluate and synthesize all relevant primary studies and "pre-appraised evidence (i.e., clinical guidelines, summaries, synopses, syntheses of relevant external evidence)" (Melnyk, Gallagher-Ford, Long, & Fineout-Overholt, 2014, p. 11);
3. integrate internal evidence and a body of external evidence from both nursing and other related health fields to make patient care decisions;
4. lead interprofessional teams to apply synthesized evidence in clinical practice changes and decisions "to improve the health of individuals, groups, and populations" (Melnyk, Gallagher-Ford, Long, & Fineout-Overholt, 2014, p. 11);
5. use EBP implementation projects and management of outcomes to integrate best practices in the organization;
6. carefully measure the "processes and outcomes of evidence-based clinical decisions" (Melnyk, Gallagher-Ford, Long, & Fineout-Overholt, 2014, p. 11);
7. develop evidence-based procedures and policies;
8. collaborate with other healthcare professionals in generating research evidence;
9. mentor others in the EBP process and evidence-based decision-making;
10. use organizational and individual strategies to sustain a culture that supports EBP; and
11. "communicate best evidence to individuals, groups, colleagues, and policy makers" [Melnyk, Gallagher-Ford, Long, & Fineout-Overholt, 2014, p. 11].

Nurse leaders must utilize organizational and individual strategies that integrate and sustain evidence-based practice in organizations to ensure high-quality, safe, cost effective care and positive outcomes to individuals, groups, and populations. They must begin by assessing the organization's readiness for EBP competencies to ensure an effective plan for their implementation. Since all nurse leaders are not knowledgeable and supportive of evidence-based practice, education and support by a nurse scientist may be essential to bring them on board and show them how to include EBP competencies in their roles (Melnyk, Gallagher-Ford, Long, & Fineout-Overholt, 2014, p. 13.).

Nurse leaders must use evidence-based competencies in their daily practice and role model EBP when making decisions. They should also expect others to use evidence-based decision-making on a daily basis and mentor other nurses to become evidence-based clinicians (Melnyk, Gallagher-Ford, Long, & Fineout-Overholt, 2014, p. 13).

Nurse leaders make hiring decisions and can incorporate evidence-based competency questions in interviews to set the tone with new employees. Including EBP competencies in position descriptions and orientation programs will establish EBP expectations for job performance. Besides serving as EBP mentors themselves, nurse leaders should seek nurses who meet or exceed EBP competencies and enable them to mentor colleagues in the clinical environment (Melnyk, Gallagher-Ford, Long, & Fineout-Overholt, 2014, p. 13).

To achieve the Quadruple Aim Framework, evidence-based practice must become the standard of care in healthcare organizations and nurse leaders should lead the way to success for individuals, groups, populations, and the interprofessional team.

Research

"The arena in which Nightingale would most certainly flourish today is nursing research. She was a consummate researcher, always asking questions and seeking the answers. Research provided the foundation to move the profession forward. She both valued and refined the art of being able to make logical and factual arguments based on data collection. Much of Nightingale's research was based on direct observation—of the patient, of the nurse, of the environment, of the outcomes of care."—Selanders, 2005, p. 72

Nursing research has evolved since Nightingale's time, but observation continues to be part of today's research process. There is a distinct difference between evidence-based practice (EBP) and research. EBP integrates external evidence with internal patient data and clinician expertise while including patient preferences and values (Melnyk, Gallagher-Ford, Long, & Fineout-Overholt, 2014, p. 5).

Research generates new evidence that can be translated into evidence-based practice and quality improvement. However, it may be years before this new evidence can be implemented in clinical settings to improve care delivery and patient outcomes because of lack of knowledge and support by leaders, clinicians, and organizations to incorporate research findings in clinical practice (Melnyk, Gallagher-Ford, Long, & Fineout-Overholt, 2014, p. 6). One government agency promotes nurse scientists' role as significant in addressing health challenges addressed in the Quadruple Aim Framework.

In 1985, the U.S. Congress enacted legislation to create a nursing research center within the National Institutes of Health (NIH). This evolved into the present-day National Institute of Nursing Research (NINR) in 1993 (NINR, 2016, p. 71). The National Institute of Nursing Research has a mission that reflects the first two Quadruple Aim measures: "to promote and improve the health and quality of life of individuals, families, and communities" (NINR, 2016, p. 6). The agency conducts and supports nursing clinical research in biological and behavioral sciences about health and illness across the lifespan to develop the scientific foundation for clinical practice. NINR also offers opportunities for training nurse scientists whose research will create new evidence to enhance the health and well-being of individuals and at-risk populations in multiple settings (NINQ, 2016, p. 6). The National Institute of Nursing Research's programs address diverse topics, such as (1) symptom science research; (2) promoting health and wellness; (3) chronic disease management; (4) support for caregivers; palliative care strategies; (5) use of innovative technologies; and (6) training in nursing science (NINR, 2016, p. 6).

Exploring each of these in depth will help nurse leaders better address all Quadruple Aim measures based on a research perspective. Each program has pertinent information to validate the importance of research by nurse scientists who seek opportunities that impact the quality of life and well-being of people facing health challenges. Such challenges include (1) population diversity; (2) increases in aging population; (3) multiple chronic conditions; (4) poorly managed symptoms of people with advanced illness; and (5) inadequate attention to needs or preferences of dying individuals (NINR, 2016, p. 3).

Symptom Science Research

Symptom science research is designed to promote personalized health strategies. NINR research seeks to develop new knowledge that will improve people's lives by testing interventions to reduce the negative effects "of symptoms, such as pain, fatigue and sleep disturbance, as well as impaired cognition and disordered mood, which can occur with numerous acute and chronic illnesses and conditions" (NINR, 2016, p. 10). Nurse scientists explore human behavior and genetics to determine if biomarkers (indicators of a disease) and genomics (DNA analysis) can be used to manage symptoms and enhance wellness. Individuals are not just dealing with one symptom at a time. Many members of at-risk populations have multiple co-morbidities and suffer from adverse symptoms related to these co-morbidities. Nurse scientists collaborate with interprofessional teams to explore new knowledge that will impact symptom science. The National Institute of Nursing Research supports this interprofessional research collaboration at facilities throughout the United States including "an intramural research program on the NIH campus in Bethesda, Maryland, dedicated to improving the understanding of the underlying biological mechanisms of a range of symptoms, their effect on patients, and the biological and behavioral bases for how patients respond to interventions" (NINR, 2016, p. 11).

An example of NINR–supported research is an international study in 2014 to identify consistent symptoms in individuals with heart failure. Researchers discovered two symptom clusters common to all 720 individuals in the study. These are (1) a physical symptom cluster—dyspnea, fatigue, and difficulty climbing or walking and (2) a cognitive/emotional symptom cluster—feelings of depression, worrying, and problems with memory, judgment, thinking and language (cognitive issues). These findings indicate that these symptoms are consistent across five cultures, including the United States, and can improve early symptom recognition of heart failure (NINR, 2016, p. 12). This will enable clinicians to begin treatment earlier and avoid adverse outcomes for this at-risk population (Quadruple Aim 2).

The National Institute of Nursing Research (NINR) uses the National Institutes of Health (NIH) Symptom Science model to facilitate research by recognition of symptom identification followed by observable characteristics of the individual reacting to the environment (phenotype) and utilization of methodologies to determine disease indicators (biomarkers) for interventions. NINR will also lead a Symptom Science Center as a place where collaborative teams of researchers "can address symptom research challenges such as those posed by multiple chronic illnesses" (NINR, 2016, p. 13).

The future direction of symptom science nursing research involves "integration of biomarkers with phenotypic indicators" (NINR, 2016, p. 13). This approach "can lead to better knowledge of the underlying biological mechanisms of symptoms such as fatigue, dyspnea, impaired cognition, pain, and disordered mood, and to improved assessment and management of these symptoms among diverse populations and settings" (NINR, 2016, p. 13). This research goes beyond current clinical assessment parameters and has potential to create personalized approaches to manage symptoms in multiple disease processes. Nurse leaders can use such research findings to address Quadruple Aim 1 (improving the experience of care for individuals) and Quadruple Aim 2 (improving the experience of care for populations).

Promoting Health and Wellness

The National Institute of Nursing Research is committed to research that supports "the physical, social, behavioral, and environmental causes of illness, determinants of health, and assessment of behaviors that lead to healthy lifestyle choices" (NINR, 2016, p. 17). Illness prevention is paramount in sustaining health and wellness for at-risk individuals and populations. Research in this area uses genomes (DNA analysis) and phenotypes (observable characteristics of the individual reacting to the environment) to predict who is at risk for developing chronic conditions and disease processes. Past research has targeted prevention of HIV (human immunodeficiency virus) in multiple settings; obesity prevention; and advocating new approaches to promote health and wellness for lay caregivers of individuals with dementia (NINR, 2016, p. 17).

NINR wellness research seeks innovative approaches to attain the highest quality of health by individuals of all ages and communities. A significant aspect of this research "is building the science to understand and prevent chronic illness, improve quality of life, reduce burden for patients and informal caregivers across the spectrum of diseases or conditions, and eliminate health disparities" (NINR, 2016, p. 17). This is a challenge that NINR believes can enhance the scientific basis for federal agencies "to improve health outcomes and health services, and reduce the burden of illness on patients and families" (NINR, 2016, p. 18). Nurse scientists collaborate with at-risk populations and minorities in community settings to develop innovative interventions that stimulate healthy behaviors and reduce incidence of chronic conditions. An example of this is a randomized control trial about healthy lifestyle promotion in high school students. The teacher in the study incorporated an intervention program in a health education class to develop social skills, healthy behaviors, academic accomplishments, and better physical health with positive results (NINR, 2016, p. 19). Replication of this study would determine if the results can be translated to other high school settings, but it shows how nurse scientists can collaborate with community members (teacher) to address population health issues.

Future NINR research to promote health and wellness by illness prevention will

1. use advances in multiple scientific arenas, including data science "to develop interventions to promote health and wellness that are leading-edge, effective, and translatable to clinical practice" (NINR, 2016, p. 21);
2. assess how the environment, nutrition, and physical activity impact "the prevention, development, and trajectory of communicable and non-communicable illnesses and acute trauma—with a particular emphasis on sex and gender differences and health disparities" (NINR, 2016, p. 21);
3. encourage interprofessional, collaborative initiatives led by nurses to use "innovative and sustainable strategies to prevent chronic conditions across the lifespan and in underrepresented minority populations" (NINR, 2016, p. 21);
4. establish social and personal approaches that can promote health and prevent illness at all ages; and
5. use diverse research methods "such as community-based participatory research and participatory action research to determine the most feasible and effective biobehavioral interventions to reduce or eliminate health disparities" (NINR, 2016, p. 21).

Nurse leaders can use research on health and wellness promotion to examine innovative approaches to Quadruple Aim 1 (improving the experience of care for individuals); Quadruple Aim 2 (improving the care of populations); and Quadruple Aim 3 (reducing the per capita cost of care and the burden on individuals and populations).

Chronic Disease Management

Many individuals (nearly 50 percent of adults) in the United States have one or more chronic diseases that adversely affect their quality of life. Such chronic illnesses also adversely impact healthcare costs nationally with more than 85 percent of costs at least partially related to chronic diseases (NINR, 2016, p. 22). These diseases do not only harm the individuals with these diagnoses. They also affect families, caregivers, communities, and society. The National Institute of Nursing Research promotes research that encourages active participation of individuals and families in self-management that "encompasses health strategies that allow an individual and their healthcare provider to adapt treatments to individual circumstances by accounting for social, cultural, economic, and emotional factors that can influence their health and quality of life" (NINR, 2016, p. 22).

An example of such research is exploring practical and innovative technologies, including electronic health records that are interactive to help clinicians and "individuals with multiple chronic conditions who must manage complex medication regimens" (NINR, 2016, p. 22). Research interventions in this area do not always have to include technology. One study demonstrated improved clinical outcomes for elderly individuals with chronic conditions by using nursing coordinated care and a medication pillbox which the elders used to correctly administer medications (NINR, 2016, p. 23). It is important to remember that individuals of all ages may have chronic conditions, such as asthmatic children and teenagers. Research must encompass all age groups as well as multiple chronic diseases.

Future research directions by the National Institute of Nursing Research to improve quality of life and health for individuals with chronic conditions include

1. delineating processes to influence self-management success for co-morbidities in various settings. This incorporates "the examination of mediators and moderators of self-management that impact adherence to treatment and sustainability or that impact interventions" (NINR, 2016, p. 25);

2. promoting health and well-being in daily activities and reducing adverse outcomes by assessing the "effects of multicomponent interventions integrating environmental factors, caregivers, and other healthcare professionals (e.g., occupational therapy, physical therapy, informatics)" (NINR, 2016, p. 25);

3. integrating social determinants of health and the individual's decision-making, health status, and infirmity "in interventions to activate access to resources to maintain health and quality of life" (NINR, 2016, p. 25);

4. investigating and utilizing "innovative technologies, devices, and biobehavioral interventions to assist in monitoring and promoting health and improving access to healthcare in those with chronic conditions" (NINR, 2016, p. 25); and

5. using methods from data science to confirm current "self-management measures, including available cohorts of existing data, to predict self-management intervention outcomes across multiple chronic conditions and in large samples" (NINR, 2016, p. 25).

Such research results will be invaluable to nurse leaders who are collaborating with other nurses and multiple disciplines to address Quadruple Aim 1 (improving the experience of care for individuals) and Quadruple Aim 2 (improving the care of populations).

Support for Caregivers/Palliative Care Strategies

The National Institute of Nursing Research is charged by NIH to lead end-of-life research that will help individuals, informal caregivers, families, and the healthcare team manage advanced illness and plan to meet end-of-life care needs. Since palliative care is essential for quality of life at all stages of serious illness, NINR focuses its efforts on "issues such as: relieving symptoms and suffering; enhancing communication between patients, families, and clinicians; and understanding decision-making surrounding care of advanced illness at the end of life" (NINR, 2016, p. 26).

To coordinate research on palliative care and end-of-life issues, NINR created the Office of End-of-Life and Palliative Care Research (OEPCR). OEPCR's research focuses on all age groups and includes families and non-medical caregivers as well as the affected individuals. Their priority is to discover new knowledge that can be used by these individuals and members of the healthcare team "to manage the complex experiences of advanced symptoms and mitigate the effects of advanced illness on the health and well-being of the individual as well as informal caregivers" (NINR, 2016, p. 27). OEPCR also studies interventions that will encourage individuals and their caregivers to make decisions about care that honor the wishes and values of the person with advanced illness. NINR is collaborating with multidisciplinary researchers from more than 60 organizations across the United States in a palliative care research cooperative "to develop scientifically based methods that lead to meaningful evidence for improving the quality of life of individuals with advanced and/or potentially life-limiting illnesses and their caregivers" (NINR, 2016, p. 28). Another example of NINR/OEPCR supported research related to palliative care and quality of health is a multicenter study where researchers addressed the safety of discontinuing statin therapy for individuals with advanced illness. There were no significant differences in mortality when statins were discontinued. These individuals also stated that their quality of life and healthcare costs improved without statin use. These results may impact efficacy of statin use in advanced illness as treatment options are discussed between the individuals and their healthcare providers (NINR, 2016, p. 28).

NINR also developed information sources for clinicians, scientists, and the public about palliative care and end-of-life care. The first of these was "The Science of Compassion: Future Directions in End-of-Life and Palliative Care," a three-day national summit in 2011 which was attended by nearly 1,000 "scientists, palliative and end-of-life care health professionals, educators, policy analysts, members of professional organizations, and members of the public" (NINR, 2016, p. 29). The summit included multiple sessions (e.g., town hall, plenary sessions, breakout sessions, and a poster session) where participants could discuss research from multiple studies to improve the quality of life for individuals with advanced illness (NINR, 2016, p. 29).

The second outreach initiative was the "Palliative Care: Conversations Matter Campaign" that was designed to "raise awareness of pediatric palliative care and to facilitate conversations about palliative care among healthcare providers, children living with a serious illness, and their families" (NINR, 2016, p. 29). After obtaining input from stakeholders, NINR developed a two-phased campaign. Phase one focused on informing healthcare providers and phase two focused on children and families by providing resources for both groups to use in talking with each other (NINR, 2016, p. 30).

The third outreach initiative was NINR's End-of-Life Module with research-based health information presented online in clear, easy to read content for older adults and their caregivers. This module is available on NIHSeniorHealth.gov and provides essential information that individuals and caregivers can use in planning and decision-making for end-of-life care (NINR, 2016, p. 30).

Future NINR research priorities for palliative and end-of-life care reflect "The Science of Compassion" and include

1. designing tactics that will enhance "integrated and coordinated care transitions, differential interventions, and treatments to improve patient-centered outcomes of hospice and palliative care across diverse care settings, populations, and cultural contexts" (NINR, 2016, p. 31);

2. delineating causes based on theory "that underlie multidimensional and complex issues and choices in end-of-life and palliative care" (NINR, 2016, p. 31);

3. creating the most effective approaches "to screen, assess, monitor, and treat the met and unmet end-of-life and palliative care needs of individuals with serious advanced illness and their families" (NINR, 2016, p. 31);

4. designing and implementing research interventions or treatments "that best address the needs of underserved, disadvantaged, and diverse populations across the care continuum" (NINR, 2016, p. 31); and

5. determining how advanced symptoms display palliative traits "with the goal of developing personalized targeted interventions to alleviate or manage symptoms" (NINR, 2016, p. 31).

Nurse leaders must understand what research is being done in palliative and end-of-life care and use scientifically-based interventions to address Quadruple Aim 1 (improving the experience of care for individuals); Quadruple Aim 2 (improving the care of populations); and Quadruple Aim 3 (reduce per capita cost of healthcare) to benefit individuals with advanced illness and members of at-risk populations while reducing costs for them.

Use of Innovative Technologies

The National Institute of Nursing Research supports research to develop innovative technologies in healthcare that will benefit underserved individuals and at-risk populations. This research encompasses "rapid advances in data science, genomic and molecular research, as well as devices and software to improve health" (NINR, 2016, p. 33). For example, a nurse-led team studied if embedding intelligent sensors in the apartments of a senior living community would detect pertinent health changes in residents. Behavioral changes outside normal activity alerted nurse clinicians on site and health changes were addressed earlier. Researchers in another study designed an ankle exoskeleton that is light and uses no power to help individuals walk more efficiently and use less energy. This prototype may be useful with further testing for older adults or those recovering from injury (NINR, 2016, p. 34).

Researchers in another study created a decision support tool that can integrate with hospital electronic health records in a three-hospital academic health system to identify patients requiring post-acute care. Findings showed a 33 percent reduction in 30-day readmissions and a 37 percent reduction in 60-day readmissions resulting in reduced hospital costs (NINR, 2016, p. 34). Using innovative technology to improve health of underserved at-risk populations is a newer field of research and NINR's future priorities include

1. determining what aspects of innovative, evidence-based interventions can be "easily tailored to diverse population groups across healthcare settings" (NINR, 2016, p. 35);

2. promoting interprofessional research "by building partnerships with technical developers (e.g., engineers and designers) and communities to design and test new technologies in various settings" (NINR, 2016, p. 35);

3. expanding the utilization of innovative technologies with cultural and community input that promotes "positive health behaviors and management of chronic conditions across conditions, communities, and ages" (NINR, 2016, p. 35); and

4. investigating multiple technological approaches "to improve the cultural congruence of health interventions and support real-time clinical decisions to improve health" (NINR, 2016, p. 35).

Nurse leaders are also using diverse technology in their daily work (e.g., data collection tools, electronic health records, smart devices). They must appreciate research results like those described above and adopt evidence-based technological interventions to address Quadruple Aim 1 (improving the experience of care for individuals); Quadruple Aim 2 (improving the care of populations); and Quadruple Aim 3 (reducing per capita cost of healthcare).

Training in Nursing Science

The National Institute of Nursing Research is committed to creating proficient nurse scientists who will contribute to innovative research methodologies that impact the health and well-being of individuals and populations while using interventions that are cost-effective and efficient. NINR has several programs to train future nurse scientists. These programs include

1. National Research Service Awards (NRSA) offering "individual and institutional predoctoral, postdoctoral, and senior fellowships" (NINR, 2016, p. 38);

2. Career Development Awards providing time and support "for an intensive, supervised career development experience leading to research independence" (NINR, 2016, p. 38);

3. NINR Summer Genetics Institute offering a summer training program that includes "genetics methodology into research on symptom management" (NINR, 2016, p. 38);

4. Symptom Methodologies Boot Camp which is a one-week intensive summer workshop addressing relevant symptoms by using "data science methods, measurement, treatments, genetics, and omics, with the goal of increasing the research capability of graduate students and faculty" (NINR, 2016, p. 38); and

5. NINR Graduate Partnerships Program (GPP) which is a doctoral fellowship program for nursing students who plan to be nurse

researchers. GPP fellows complete a dissertation research project "in pathophysiological mechanisms related to symptoms and symptom management, health promotion, disease prevention, tissue injury, and genetics" (NINR, 2016, p. 38).

NINR realizes that future nurse scientists must be well prepared to lead interprofessional and interdisciplinary teams and create new evidence that will address the strategies previously described (e.g., symptom science; promoting health and wellness; improving quality of life for individuals with chronic conditions; palliative and end-of-life care, and using innovative technology to improve health). Diversity is essential for nurse scientists who will lead teams and within the research workforce. NINR continues to develop the nurse scientists of the future.

Nurse leaders cannot all attend available NINR programs for research careers, but they must be able to understand research concepts and methodology, how to interpret data results, and if conclusions validate the hypothesis or research question. Each study should be read critically to determine if it is valid (measures what it should) and reliable (produces stable and consistent results). As mentioned earlier, it may take years for research findings to be incorporated in evidence-based practice and quality improvement. Replication (repeating the study in another setting) may be needed to validate the initial results. Research is not a rapid process, but well-conducted research is vital to progress in nursing and healthcare. Nurse leaders must champion sound research that that will help them and other healthcare team members address the Quadruple Aim Framework in their area(s) of employment.

Diversity

"The one gleam of comfort through it all was the rush of all English-speaking people, in all climates and in all longitudes, who have contributed every penny they could so ill spare. In this awful war, all, all have given—every man, woman, and child above pauperism. I have been so touched to receive from places I had never even heard of, but which it would take me a day to enumerate,—from poor hard-working negro congregations of all kinds, Puritan chapels in my own dear hills, National Schools, Factories, London dissenting congregations without a single rich member, London ragged schools who having nothing to give, gave up their only feast in the year that the money might be sent to the orphans in the war 'who want it more than we."—Florence Nightingale (Cook, 1913b, p. 198)

The Franco-German War of 1870–1871 was the occasion of the above quotation. When people around the world heard that Nightingale needed help for people in the war zone who were in desperate need, the response was phenomenal and illustrates that diversity can exemplify unity in a cause everyone can support. Nightingale inspired loyalty in even those she never met because her example was universally known and revered (Cook, 1913b).

Today, the National Institute of Nursing Research continues to promote diversity in its nurse scientists and interprofessional/interdisciplinary teams to reflect the individuals and populations in their studies. It is important to remember that diversity encompasses age, gender, ethnicity, race, religion, and sexual orientation (Avalon, Washington, & Harris-Cater, 2017, p. 49). Nurse scientists are obligated to protect the rights of research subjects, especially "vulnerable groups, including children, cognitively impaired persons, economically or educationally disadvantaged persons, fetuses, older adults, patients, pregnant women, prisoners, and underserved populations" (ANA, 2015, pp. 10–11). Since the United States population is not homogenous, diversity within research teams will enable them to relate to the individuals and populations they are studying.

Diversity goes beyond research settings into clinical practice environments now and in the future. The United States is a multilingual and multiracial society where cultural sensitivity, cultural competence, and inclusion are vital to the health and well-being of diverse community members. Today's registered nurse population does not reflect that of the United States. According to U.S. Census Bureau data in September 2018, population demographics were

62% (197 million) White;
16.9% (53.9 million) Hispanic;
12.6% (40.2 million) Black;
5.2% (16.6 million) Asian;
2.3% (7.2 million) Mixed; and
1% (3.27 million) Other [Race and Ethnicity in the United States, 2018].

The racial/ethnic composition of registered nurses in 2017 was

71.34% (2,458,594 RNs) White;
6.81% (234,729 RNs) Hispanic;
10.38% (357,888 RNs) Black;
9.08% (313,230 RNs) Asian;
1.76% (60,786 RNs) Two or more races;
0.21% (7,428 RNs) Other;

0.05% (1,766 RNs) Native Hawaiian or Pacific Islander; and 0.33% (11,665 RNs) American Indian or Alaska Native [Campaign for Action, 2019].

Nurse leaders must ensure that cultural sensitivity and cultural competence are attributes of nurses caring for diverse individuals and populations who may have special healthcare needs. Identifying such needs is essential, particularly if they adversely impact certain segments of the population. The Centers for Disease Control and Prevention (CDC) has sponsored interventions to reduce health disparities in specific races and cultures. Such interventions incorporated research findings with evidence-based practice for diverse populations including the following.

1. Diabetes prevention and health promotion in Alaska Native and American Indian communities—Early in this decade tribal adults were 2.1 times more likely to be diagnosed with diabetes than non–Hispanic white adults. Teenagers between 15–19 and young adults 18–34 had increased risk of diabetes, particularly if they were obese. Many tribes ate a high-fiber diet and available land did not always support food and agriculture systems. In 2008, the CDC created a five-year Traditional Foods Project for access to traditional foods and support for health promotion. A sixth year of funding was requested in 2014 and analysis of results showed that (1) reverence for the land contributed to sustainable food systems; (2) tribes are working to revive traditional foods; (3) traditional knowledge about the land helped rebuild food systems; (4) traditional values about health related to cultural values; (5) elders taught youth and connected socially with them; (6) traditional foods created conversations about health; (7) education about traditional foods engaged all generations; (8) communities used multiple avenues to plan strategies to address their needs; and (9) programs continued even after the end of the initiative in 2014 by seeking other funding sources and alliances (Satterfield, DeBruyn, Santos, Alonzo,, & Frank, 2016);

2. Community asthma initiative to reduce disparities and improve health outcomes for children with asthma—Based on a study in Boston, Black and Hispanic children who live in poverty are hospitalized more frequently for poorly controlled asthma than White children in the same age group. The Community Asthma Initiative (CAI) enables nurses and health workers to make home visits and conduct community-based case management for asthma. Since many families did not speak English at home, CAI hired Spanish-speaking community health workers to work with families. The agency also partnered

with other organizations caring for children and addressed housing violations that affected the health of children with asthma. CAI and its civic partners addressed social determinants of health to ensure environmental safety for these children ranging from two to 18 years. A longitudinal study evaluated progress for each enrolled child over a seven-year period. After 12 months, participants had a 79 percent decrease in hospitalizations for asthma; a 56 percent decrease in ED visits; a 42 percent decrease in missed schooldays; a 46 percent decrease in missed workdays for parents and guardians; and a 29 percent decrease in limited activity days (Woods, et al., 2016, p. 14). The CAI initiative contains "all components of the chronic care model, including addressing patient safety, cultural competency, care coordination, community policies, and case management, for improving the care of patients and families living with a chronic illness" (Woods, et al., 2016, p. 16);

3. Evidence-based interventions to address disparities in colorectal cancer screening—Although colorectal cancer is the second leading cause of death in U.S. cancers and screening is recommended for adults from 50–75 years, racial/ethnic minorities often are not screened. These populations lack health insurance, are less educated, and live at marginal economic levels. The CDC's Colorectal Cancer Control Program (CRCCP) began in 2009 to increase screening for these populations to 80 percent. The highest incidence of colorectal cancer in the United States occurs in Alaska Native persons who also have twice the mortality rate of White individuals. CRCCP partnered with the Alaska Native Tribal Health Consortium and its healthcare facilities to ensure that electronic health records contained information about colorectal cancer screening. This data was supplemented by nurse navigators who educated and encouraged Alaska Natives to be screened. Annual screening data was maintained and analyzed to determine rates in this adult population. Initial results showed that compliance by Alaska Native adults was 50.9 percent The latest statistics (2012) showed that 59.8 percent of these adults had been screened in compliance with CRCCP recommendations. In 2011 a similar situation occurred in the State of Washington where minority populations who were not insured and lived at the federal poverty level also lacked compliance with recommended colorectal cancer screening Baseline date showed 24 percent compliance. Evidence-based interventions mirrored those for Alaska Natives and compliance increased to 48 percent by 2014. Although online reminders and information is useful, multiple interventions (e.g., patient reminders, provider reminders,

nurse navigators) are essential for successful screening (Joseph, Redwood, DeGroff, & Butler, 2016).

4. Reducing health disparities to eliminate Hepatitis A virus in the United States—The Hepatitis A virus (HAV) is highly infectious and spreads from contaminated food and water, inadequate sanitation, and poor living conditions. Major racial/ethnic groups affected are Hispanics, Blacks, and American Indians/Alaska Natives. The CDC Office of Minority Health and Health Equity chose vaccination as an intervention to reduce/eliminate the Hepatitis A virus in at-risk populations. This has expanded to include all children beginning at 12–23 months of age. This intervention decreased the incidence of Hepatitis A virus in each racial/ethnic group to less than one case per 100,000 people eliminating most health disparities related to HAV. However, in recent years the number of vaccinated adults has declined and the gap between vaccinated children and unvaccinated adults is a emerging health disparity that will require new intervention strategies to eliminate Hepatitis A virus in the future (Murphy, et al., 2016).

5. Use of an evidence-based HIV prevention intervention for high-risk men who have sex with other men—Same sex behavior without condom use increases incidence of HIV infection in Black and Hispanic/Latino men. This population has significantly lower HIV testing rates and medical treatment of this diagnosis. This can be related to their concern about others' perceptions about their sexual orientation which may be manifested in discrimination by providers, lack of insurance coverage, and inadequate access to health services that are welcoming to homosexuals and bisexuals. The CDC's National HIV Surveillance System and Medical Monitoring Project supported use of Personalized Cognitive Counseling (PCC) which is an evidence-based behavioral intervention to reduce anal sex without condom use by HIV-negative men who have sex with men (MSM). This initiative begins with a short counseling session with these at-risk individuals that covers (1) individual's recent unforgettable experience of unprotected anal intercourse (UAI); (2) completion of PCC questionnaire by individual; (3) counselor-guided discussion about individual's feelings about experience in #1; (4) discussion about self-justifying comments; and (5) discussion about what individual will do in the future. This is followed by HIV testing and the session lasts no more than 50 minutes. Project ECHO, funded by the CDC adapted the PCC for use with high-risk populations in San Francisco. Adaptation focused on substance use and self-justifications. Two randomized trials showed that PCC was effective with non-substance using Black, Hispanic, Asian,

and mixed-race participants reporting a 59 percent reduction in the number of unprotected anal intercourse. PCC substance-using participants also reported a 46 percent reduction in alcohol intoxication and a 74 percent reduction in the number of unprotected anal intercourse events with use of methamphetamine. Men who have sex with men are still at greater risk for HIV infection and the adapted PCC is a behavioral, evidence-based intervention that can reduce substance-use and personal risk behaviors by reducing health disparities for these individuals (Herbst, et al., 2016).

6. Interventions to reduce HIV disparities among immigrant Hispanic/Latino men—Hispanics/Latinos are affected by HIV, AIDS, and sexually transmitted diseases (STDs) more than non–Hispanic Whites. The CDC Office of Minority Health and Health Equity sought an evidence-based program to reduce HIV disparities in this population and used "a community-based participatory research (CBPR) partnership" (Rhodes, Leichliter, Sun, & Bloom, 2016, p. 51). This partnership developed an intervention in Spanish to promote condom use and HIV and STD testing in Hispanic/Latino men by using lay health advisors and socialization in soccer teams used for recreation. This initiative was titled "HoMBReS: Hombres Manteniendo Bienestar y Relaciones Saludables (Men Maintaining Wellbeing and Healthy Relationships)" (Rhodes, Leichliter, Sun, & Bloom, 2016, p. 52). Lay health navigators (Navegantes) were team members who were trained to communicate comfortably and offer sound advice. They also were required to have time for the role and transportation to attend team functions. The Navegantes also served as community advocates. This intervention increased condom usage and was recognized as a best practice by the CDC. Self-reporting also showed increased HIV testing. It has been replicated in another community successfully. Subsequently, an advanced intervention HoMBReS Por un Cambio (Men for Change) used DVDs for additional training for Navegantes and for them to use with teammates. It also used temas del mes (themes of the month) to guide activities. These themes can include living with HIV and accessing public health services for HIV and STD testing. HoMBReS has been revised for use with transgender and men having sex with men (MSM) populations. This successful initiative may be feasible for other health issues in other populations. (Rhodes, Leichliter, Sun, & Bloom, 2016).

7. Using economic, policy, and structural strategies to prevent violence in high-risk youth and communities—Homicide as the cause of death is #1 in Black youths ages 10–24 years; #2 in Hispanic youths;

#3 in American Indian/Alaska Native youths; and #4 in Asian/Pacific Islander youths. Significant research has been done to prevent violence for youths in minority populations. However, interventions have not addressed the community at large. Community risk factors are variable, but must be addressed for interventions to succeed. The CDC's Division of Violence Prevention focuses on community strategies to reduce or prevent violence. The CDC Office of Minority Health and Health Equity analyzed three interventions in different communities to determine effective strategies to reduce violence-related disparities in these settings. The first intervention was creating Business Improvement Districts (BIDs) by investing resources from local businesses to improve the service area. Longitudinal results showed significant reduction in violence where BIDs exist. In Los Angeles, BIDs "were associated with a 12 percent reduction in robberies (one type of violent crime) and an 8 percent reduction of violent crime overall" (Massetti & David-Ferdon, 2016, pp. 58–59). The second intervention restricted the sale of single-serve alcohol by convenience stores. After six months, the policy was reversed due to opposition by grocery owners. Researchers were able to evaluate the impact of the policy by tracking injuries pre- and post-restrictions. Transport by ambulance of violently-injured youths decreased significantly when the policy was effective from 19.6 to zero per 1,000 population. This rate increased to 11.4 per 1,000 in the 18 months after the policy was rescinded. The third intervention was Safe Streets where neighborhoods were mobilized to make violence unacceptable and promote positive community events. In one neighborhood this intervention resulted in a 56 percent reduction in homicides and a 34 percent reduction in nonfatal shootings after two years. In other communities, results were mixed. One other community saw decrease of 26 percent for homicides and 22 percent for nonfatal shootings. Another community had no changes in homicides and a reduction of 34 percent in nonfatal shootings. The fourth community showed 2.7 times increase in homicide and a 44 percent decrease in nonfatal shootings. That community had high rates of gang activity and only 18 months of data are available. The Centers for Disease Control and Prevention (CDC) continues to evaluate community strategies like these to explore their potential to reduce health disparities related to violence for youths (Massetti & David-Ferdon, 2016).

These examples illustrate how research and evidence-based practice can reduce health disparities in at-risk populations of all ages and ethnicity.

Nurse leaders must ensure that care is culturally sensitive and culturally competent. They also must create a culturally sensitive environment for nurses and other healthcare team members from minority populations. Nurses will not mirror the changes in the population of the United States within a short period of time, but adding diverse team members will help nurses address disparities that adversely impact the success of the Quadruple Aim.

The Standards of Practice for nurses is relevant for nurse leaders in this context.

1. Standard 1. Assessment—"The registered nurse collects pertinent data and information relative to the healthcare consumer's health or the situation" (ANA, 2015, p. 53). This data is not limited to physical findings. The consumer is also unique based on cultural, spiritual, environmental, sexual, gender, psychosocial, and economic status. The healthcare consumer makes choices based on his/her values, beliefs, literacy, and cultural background. Family dynamics will also impact the consumer's choices about health and wellness. The nurse must keep the consumer's care preferences upfront in the assessment process (ANA, 2015, p. 53),

2. Standard 2. Diagnosis—"The registered nurse analyzes assessment data to determine actual or potential diagnoses, problems, and issues" (ANA, 2015, p. 55). The nurse must collaborate with the healthcare consumer to develop goals that address risks and barriers to health and wellness "which may include but are not limited to interpersonal, systematic, cultural, or environmental circumstances" (ANA, 2015, p. 55).

3. Standard 3. Outcomes Identification—"The registered nurse identifies expected outcomes for a plan individualized to the healthcare consumer or the situation" (ANA, 2015, p. 57). Using information from assessment and diagnosis, the nurse determines expected outcomes that are culturally sensitive and "collaborates with the healthcare consumer to define expected outcomes integrating the healthcare consumer's culture, values, and ethical considerations" (ANA, 2015, p. 57). The nurse uses these expected outcomes to coordinate care with the healthcare team.

4. Standard 4. Planning—"The registered nurse develops a plan that prescribes strategies to attain expected, measurable outcomes" (ANA, 2015, p. 59). The nurse uses evidence-based strategies to address the healthcare consumer's needs based on the three previous steps. The nurse, healthcare consumer, and interprofessional team partner to

develop "an individualized, holistic, evidence-based plan" (ANA, 2015, p. 59).

5. Standard 5. Implementation—"The registered nurse implements the identified plan" (ANA, 2015, p. 61). The nurse partners with the healthcare consumer and the interprofessional team to implement evidence-based strategies to achieve identified outcomes. The nurse also "provides culturally congruent, holistic care that focuses on the healthcare consumer and addresses and advocates for the needs of diverse populations across the lifespan" (ANA, 2015, p. 61).

6. Standard 5A. Coordination of Care—"The registered nurse coordinates care delivery" (ANA, 2015, p. 63). The nurse encourages the healthcare consumer in self-care to promote health and wellness and "communicates with the healthcare consumer, interprofessional team, and community-based resources to effect safe transitions in continuity of care" (ANA, 2015, p. 63).

7. Standard 5B. Health Teaching and Health Promotion—"The registered nurse employs strategies to promote health and a safe environment" (ANA, 2015, p. 65). The nurse guides the healthcare consumer to information about health and disease prevention. The nurse "uses health promotion and health teaching methods in collaboration with the healthcare consumer's values, beliefs, health practices, developmental level, learning needs, readiness and ability to learn, language preference, spirituality, culture, and socioeconomic status" (ANA, 2015, p. 65).

8. Standard 6. Evaluation—"The registered nurse evaluates progress toward attainment of goals and outcomes" (ANA, 2015, p. 66). The nurse partners with the healthcare consumer and other members of the healthcare team and family to evaluate the effectiveness of implemented actions. The nurse "determines, in partnership with the healthcare consumer and other stakeholders, the patient-centeredness, effectiveness, efficiency, safety, timeliness, and equitability of the strategies in relation to the responses to the plan and attainment of outcomes" (ANA, 2015, p. 66).

Adherence to these standards and attention to the needs of diverse individuals and populations is essential for nurse leaders at all levels to provide culturally congruent and sensitive care and successfully address the Quadruple Aim Framework.

Political Savvy and Legislative Advocacy

> "We are trying to reduce chaos into shape. It is three years today since I first felt what an awful wreck, I had

got myself into. I interfering with government affairs; and the captain of my ship, without whom I should never have done it, dying and leaving me, a woman, in charge. What nonsense people do talk, to be sure, about people finding themselves in suitable positions and looking out for congenial work. I am sure if any body in all the world is most unsuited for writing and official work, it is I. And yet I have done nothing else for seven years but write regulations."—Florence Nightingale (Cook, 1913b, p. 59)

Nightingale wrote this in 1864 when she was serving as an advisor to the War Office for the Army. She refers to her friend and mentor, Sidney Herbert, who was Secretary of State prior to his death. Her engagement in the political life of the British Empire would continue many years and her influence on the politicians of her era was considerable (Cook, 1913b).

Today, nurse leaders must also demonstrate political savvy and legislative advocacy if they are to achieve the Quadruple Aim Framework in their professional and personal endeavors. The word "politics" means different things to different people. For some individuals, it invokes dread and a negative perception. For others, it is something to tolerate in work and daily life. Still others enjoy organizational and/or legislative politics as challenges leading to success. Nurse leaders must be in the last group if they and the Quadruple Aim are to succeed.

Political Savvy

Political savvy is a journey that begins with social thinking. Social thinking is not social skills. An individual can be socially skilled without being politically savvy. Social skills can be defined "as the ability to effectively adapt our social behavior around others according to the situation, what we know about the people in that situation, and what our own needs are" (Winner & Crooke, 2011, p. 2). Social thinking "is how we think about our own and others' minds" (Winner & Crooke, 2011, p. 2). This is the foundation of our social skills and requires the individual nurse leader to gain insight into his/her own thoughts about others to be sensitive to other people in multiple situations. This includes direct and indirect interactions. Nurse leaders who master this skill will adapt their behavior to build relationships where both parties are satisfied with the end result (Winner & Crooke, 2011).

It is important to remember that the word "politics" is neither good or bad. It is simply a fact of life in healthcare and other organizations. Attention to social thinking is a good beginning and socially astute individuals interpret their own and others' behavior accurately in social interactions. They are keen observers and able to identify with others to achieve positive results (Ferris, Davidson, & Perrewé, 2005). Social astuteness sets the stage for the next step in political savvy-interpersonal influence where the individual's personal style elicits desired responses from others. This requires flexibility and adaptability in different settings and situations and success focuses on achieving results gracefully and positively. Politically savvy individuals create and use diverse networks and alliances of others who are valuable allies for both personal and professional success. They are liked and respected as well as adept at managing conflict. These individuals "possess high levels of social capital, which enhances their reputation and ability to be influential" (Ferris, Davidson, & Perrewé, 2005, p. 11). The fourth aspect of political savvy involves being perceived by others as honest, sincere, and caring. Politically savvy individuals inspire confidence and trust because they "astutely assess every situation to determine the most appropriate methods and techniques of influence to employ in that context, and then execute them to perfection" (Ferris, Davidson, & Perrewé, 2005, p. 7).

How does this work in healthcare and what can nurse leaders in multiple healthcare settings do to influence others to implement Quadruple Aim measures in their organizations? Here are ten steps to achieve the desired results by

1. knowing who the key players are in the organization (Johnson, 2017, p. 40). Titles are not always indicative of influence. Implementing Quadruple Aim measures will require organizational change and the nurse leader must observe who influences change decisions and how those individuals promote teamwork. Using the skills outlined above, the nurse leader can connect with these influential players and gain their support in making the changes necessary to incorporate Quadruple Aim measures in the organization;

2. practicing political savvy (Johnson, 2017, p. 40). Nurse leaders "must learn how decisions are made in your organization, who plays what role in the organization, and how you can promote others' interests to establish alliances that will influence organizational outcomes" (Johnson, 2017, p. 40). These outcomes will include better individual experience of care (Quadruple Aim 1); improving the health of at-risk populations (Quadruple Aim 2); reducing healthcare costs (Quadruple Aim 3); and improvement of provider work life and team vitality (Quadruple Aim 4);

3. having a seat at the table (Johnson, 2017, p. 40). Many nurse leaders are already at the decision-making table, but others (particularly

those in education and academia) may not be currently included. These nurse leaders may begin their organizational integration by volunteering for formal and informal work teams whose activities impact the organization and its bottom line. Examples include quality, risk management, infection prevention, and task forces addressing fiscal impact (e.g., readmission rates; nurse sensitive indicators; and length of stay). Remember that politically savvy individuals influence others to achieve desired results. This starts with becoming involved in interprofessional committees and groups within the organization and translates to becoming a powerful voice for Quadruple Aim measures that will benefit individuals, populations, cost reduction, and team vitality;

4. focusing on the organization's strategic initiatives (Johnson, 2017, p. 40). As nurse leaders gain visibility and influence within their organizations, they must understand and support organizational strategic initiatives. These initiatives drive the business and success of the organization. Politically savvy nurse leaders understand that Quadruple Aim measures are reflected in the organization's strategic plan and must be incorporated for the organization to succeed in its mission. It is their role to ensure that the organization's key players understand and support this inclusion;

5. developing allies (Johnson, 2017, p. 40). Developing a network of individuals was discussed earlier and such a network is essential to achieving the nurse leader's personal and professional objectives in alignment with the organization's goals. Nurse leaders always seek to expand their network as "an opportunity to explore interprofessional collaboration among multiple disciplines who are all unified for quality patient care" (Johnson, 2017, p. 40);

6. collaborating and communicating with others (Johnson, 2017, p. 40). Nurse leaders realize that multiple interactions occur informally outside formal channels and meetings. Since time is valuable, nurse leaders must be alert to others' interests if they plan to influence behavior about the Quadruple Aim. Brevity and clarity are essential as "time constraints require clear, concise descriptions about issues, possible actions, and recommended approaches" (Johnson, 2017, p. 40);

7. being a team player (Johnson, 2017, p. 41). Politically savvy nurse leaders are perceived as trustworthy, honest, and supportive of others by giving them credit for their ideas and input while they seek decisions that will benefit the organization. Implementing Quadruple Aim measures is such a decision. Nurse leaders "remember to see others' point of view, listen attentively, and advocate based on the issues" (Johnson, 2017, p. 41);

8. quantitatively measuring results (Johnson, 2017, p. 41). Implementing Quadruple Aim measures will incur initial costs from organizational changes, but the benefits will outweigh the costs. Nurse leaders must ally themselves with finance and human resource department representatives to ensure measurement of patient experience of care via HCAHPS (Quadruple Aim 1); readmission rates within 30 days of individuals with congestive heart failure in this at-risk population (Quadruple Aim 2); cost savings realized from compliance with nurse-sensitive indicators (Quadruple Aim 3); and reduced turnover costs because of improved provider work life (Quadruple Aim 4);

9. ethically playing the game (Johnson, 2017, p. 41). Politics in organizations is not negative. It is part of organizational life and nurse leaders must be honest and ethical in interactions with organization alliances and coalitions. Their ability to see the big picture and approaching situations ethically enables others to see them "as authentic and a positive force in the organization" (Johnson, 2017, p. 41); and

10. seeking self and others' professional growth (Johnson, 2017, p. 41). Politically savvy nurse leaders must mentor others to develop their knowledge, while continuing to enhance their own professional learning. As they continue to develop their own expertise in areas like the Quadruple Aim Framework, nurse leaders have an obligation to share their knowledge with others to advance the profession and healthcare (Johnson, 2017, p. 41).

Legislative Advocacy

If the Quadruple Aim Framework is to succeed in advancing healthcare in the United States, its tenets must be supported with legislation at the local, state, and federal levels. Nurse leaders must expand their political savvy to advocate for legislative reforms that will improve the experience of care for individuals (Quadruple Aim 1); improve the health of at-risk populations (Quadruple Aim 2); and reduce healthcare costs (Quadruple Aim 3). Advocacy is about collaboration, not competition, and nurse leaders must understand the legislative process, the key players, and how to navigate the road to healthcare reform to successfully address the Quadruple Aim.

The Legislative Process

The legislative process follows certain steps as a proposed bill becomes law in city councils, county boards, state legislatures, and the U.S. Congress. Most legislation occurs in Congress and state legislatures.

Step 1—Bill Introduction

A senator or representative must introduce a bill for consideration. That person becomes the sponsor and other legislators may co-sponsor the bill because they support the content or have helped prepare it. Important bills may have several co-sponsors Congress will consider four types of legislation—bills; simple resolutions; joint resolutions; and concurrent resolutions. Public bills affect the public in general and private bills affect certain individuals or private parties (USLegal, n.d.).

Step 2—Committee Referral

When a bill or resolution is introduced, it is referred to a standing committee of either the House or Senate. Major legislation is often referred to more than one committee (USLegal, n.d.).

Steps 3 and 4— Committee Action/Subcommittee Review

The bill is carefully reviewed by either the entire committee or a designated subcommittee and its chances of passage are evaluated. If more than one committee must review, the first committee must send it to the second committee, which can only act on the bill. If the second committee does not act, the bill is essentially dead. Committee approval allows the bill to continue (USLegal, n.d.).

Step 5—Mark Up

When hearings are finished, the subcommittee may make amendments and changes to the bill and send it back to the full committee for approval (Mark Up). If the bill is not reported to the full committee, it does not become law (USLegal, n.d.).

Step 6—Committee Action—Reporting the Bill

If the subcommittee sends the bill to the full committee, a review occurs about the subcommittee's recommendations. The committee may hold additional hearings or vote on its final recommendations for the House or Senate. Bills passing this stage are reported (USLegal, n.d.).

Step 7—Committee Report Publication

Now, a written report is published about "the intent and scope of the bill, its impact on existing laws, budgetary considerations, and any new taxes or tax increases that will be required by the bill" (USLegal, n.d.). This report may include hearing transcripts and committee opinions pro and con (USLegal, n.d.)

Step 8—Floor Action Scheduling

The bill is placed in chronological order on the calendar and scheduled for debate by the chamber's members. As the bill waits for debate, it may be sent to the same or another committee for reconsideration. That will eliminate any chance for the bill to receive a final vote and it will die in committee (USLegal, n.d.).

Step 9—Debate

Debate for an against the bill occurs following established procedures, including time allotted for general debate (USLegal, n.d.).

Step 10—Voting

After debate, the full membership will vote on the bill either by voice vote or roll-call (USLegal, n.d.).

Step 11—Bill Referral to the Other Chamber

If the bill is approved, it is sent to the other chamber where the process is the same as outlined above. The second chamber has the following options as it sees fit—"approve, reject, ignore, or amend the bill" (USLegal, n.d.).

Step 12—Role of Conference Committee

If the second chamber makes major changes to the bill, a conference committee of three to five members of both chambers will meet to reconcile the differences between each chamber's version of the bill. If the committee cannot come to a resolution, the bill dies. If a compromise is achieved, the conference committee prepares a conference report about the changes. Both chambers must approve this report. If they do not, the bill is sent back to the conference committee for further review (USLegal, n.d.).

Step 13—Final Action

When both chambers have approved the identical bill, it is considered enrolled and is sent to the President for signature. A signed bill becomes law when the President signs it or takes no action for 10 days while Congress is in session. If the President vetoes the bill or does not act on it for 10 days when Congress is not in their second session, the bill dies. This is called a pocket veto (USLegal, n.d.).

Step 14—Overriding the Veto

A 2/3 vote by a quorum of members of both chambers is required for the bill to become law over a presidential veto (USLegal, n.d.).

Resolutions don't require a presidential signature and simple resolutions only affect one chamber. Concurrent resolutions affect both chambers and joint resolutions are similar to a bill and may be used to amend the Constitution. Concurrent resolutions must be approved by 2/3 of both chambers and do not go to the President for approval. They are sent to the states for ratification (U.S. Congress, n.d.).

The Key Players in Healthcare Legislation

When the nurse leader understands the process outlined above for a bill to become law, he/she must know who the key players are to advocate successfully for legislative changes in healthcare. Some will be allies, others will have differing viewpoints. Here are some of the key legislative players for healthcare.

1. Legislators are elected officials who handle the bill process outlined above. Many legislators are not knowledgeable about healthcare and nurse leaders must educate them in the importance of Quadruple Aim measures in healthcare across the United States (AONL, n.d.).

2. Federal agencies' role in the legislative process has been described previously and their representatives may be allies in bills that address at-risk populations and cost-effective care (HHS.gov, 2018).

3. Public agencies are also working with clients with health and social disparities and can lend their voice to the nurse leader's in advocating for healthcare legislation (Li, Kong, Lawley, Weiss, & Pagán, 2015).

4. Professional organizations are excellent resources and many have employees as legislative liaisons who have invaluable data and expertise in navigating the healthcare legislative process (ANA Enterprise, n.d.).

5. Regulatory agencies have data about patient experience and care

delivery for populations as well as financial data that will be useful for the nurse leader in talking with legislators (Centers for Medicare and Medicaid Services, 2018).

6. Providers, such as healthcare organizations, can also contribute data and support if they are aligned with the nurse leader to promote legislation for Quadruple Aim measures (leapfrogggroup.org);

7. Payers, such as insurance providers, will provide legislative support if their costs will be reduced by healthcare legislation (Healthy-People2020 and CAPP, 2017).

8. The public will support the Quadruple Aim if they understand it and the measures benefit them (ANA, 2015).

Navigating Healthcare Reform as a Legislative Advocate

Nurse leaders who are politically savvy, understand the complex legislative process, and know the key players are prepared to advocate for healthcare reform by addressing the Quadruple Aim in legislation. Advocacy is about collaboration so the nurse leader must use his/her communication and collaboration skills to form alliances with key individuals in healthcare legislation that impacts the Quadruple Aim and benefits individuals, at-risk populations, and cost-effective care.

The Public

> "If the public choose to recognize my services and my judgment in this matter, they must leave these services and that judgment unfettered."—Florence Nightingale (Cook, 1913a, p. 269)

Florence Nightingale wrote this from the Crimea after hearing that the British public was collecting funds to recognize her service there. These contributions came from all levels of society, including the Queen and her poorest subjects. The result was the Nightingale Fund which created the first training school for nurses in England (Cook, 1913a).

Today, of all the key players in healthcare legislation, public support is vital. They are healthcare consumers and their input may often be ignored by others. However, they are integral members of the interprofessional team and their needs are paramount. Social determinants of health and health disparities are often more important to members of the public than complying with the medical plan. If forced to choose between food and medication, they will spend meager funds on food for themselves and their families. Nurse leaders realize the importance of public perceptions of care as they advocate for legislation to protect the public's access to healthcare and availability of cost-effective health services (HealthyPeople2020). Partnership and collaboration with recipients of healthcare services enhances their willingness to support legislators who sponsor legislation that positively impacts their home and health situation (Quadruple Aim 1).

Payers

Payers require a different approach by politically savvy nurse leaders seeking to obtain their support for healthcare legislation that benefits at-risk populations (Quadruple Aim 2). Payers want their clients (members of the public) to stay healthy because health and well-being result in reduced payouts by insurers. Nurse leaders can use this information to collaborate with payers for legislation that will reduce per capita health costs (Quadruple Aim 3).

Providers

Providers in diverse healthcare settings have a vested interest in all four Quadruple Aim Measures. HCAHPS data reflects individual patient perceptions of care (Quadruple Aim 1) and can result in reduced reimbursement to healthcare facilities (Quadruple Aim 3). Care of at-risk populations (Quadruple Aim 2) also affects reimbursement when readmissions occur less than 30 days post-discharge. Concerns about provider work life (Quadruple Aim 4) also affect absenteeism and turnover costs. The politically savvy nurse leader can leverage these issues to gain support from providers for legislation that will positively impact these issues.

Regulatory Agencies

The role of regulatory agencies is different from the three groups above. Healthcare regulatory agencies work to improve healthcare quality, safety, and effectiveness. Since older adults comprise an at-risk population, the Centers for Medicare and Medicaid Services (CMS) seeks to ensure quality, cost-effective, and efficient care for this population. Both agencies are excellent resources for data that politically savvy nurse leaders can use in conversations with legislators to enhance support for legislation that positively affects individuals, at-risk populations and cost-effective, cost-efficient care.

Professional Organizations

Professional nursing organizations, such as the American Nurses Association (ANA) Enterprise, frequently have advocacy departments to address state and federal legislation that impacts the safety, well-being, and health of individuals and at-risk populations. These individuals and organizations are excellent resources, both in access to relevant data and in knowledge about how to navigate the legislative process (ANA Enterprise, n.d.). Their input and advice will be invaluable to politically savvy nurse leaders who are new to legislative advocacy.

Public Agencies

The local health department is an excellent resource for the politically savvy nurse leader. This public agency is tasked with promoting the health, safety, and well-being of all area residents. If the nurse leader is advocating for local or state legislation that will impact these residents, the health department has valuable data about health disparities and can access the state health department for additional resources. Since the impact is local, citizen advocates can coordinate a team approach to legislators about proposed Quadruple Aim legislation (Li, Kong, Lawley, Weiss, & Pagán, 2015).

Federal Agencies

Federal agencies, such as the National Institutes of Health (NIH), the Agency for Healthcare Research & Quality (AHRQ), and the Centers for Disease Control (CDC), are also active participants in healthcare. The politically savvy nurse leader can consult and communicate with these agencies for information about disparities that affect the health and well-being of individuals and populations. All three agencies are part of the Department of Health & Human Services and are charged with protecting Americans' health and well-being. Their mission reflects the Quadruple Aim Framework, making them allies to cultivate as the nurse leader advocates for legislation that promotes the health and well-being of individuals and populations with cost-effective, efficient services (HHS.gov, 2018).

Legislators

Legislators are elected on a local, state, or national level for varying terms of office. The first step in contacting legislators is to discover who represents the district or the state. The state nurses' association can connect the nurse leader with the correct legislator(s). It's important to remember that every legislator is not a healthcare expert and must rely on staff members, constituent input, and outside expertise to effectively represent the electorate. Since the legislator's time is limited, the politically savvy nurse leader will also want to develop a relationship with trusted staffers who can support the proposed legislation. Remember that advocacy is about collaboration and developing a relationship with the legislator(s) will facilitate that collaboration (AONL, n.d.).

Whether the nurse leader uses email, social media, or call/direct visit depends on the urgency of the issue and its complexity. Here are tips for using each of these avenues.

Email

1. If the nurse leader has recently interacted with the legislator or staffer, remind the person to make the message more personal.
2. Quickly come to the point. The recipient's time is valuable.
3. Stick to one or two issues and be clear and concise.
4. Attach any additional material and a telephone number for any questions.
5. Share a personal experience.
6. Use real-life examples to describe the issue [AONL, n.d.].

Social Media

Most legislators have Facebook and Twitter accounts. The nurse leader should check these sites to see if the legislator holds the same views about the Quadruple Aim and proposed legislation. If this is the case, the nurse leader can participate in discussion and share relevant information (AONL, n.d.).

Calling or Direct Meeting

Politically savvy nurse leaders should

1. use these approaches for urgent issues;
2. come to the point quickly;
3. prepare for the discussion with facts and talking points;
4. anticipate answering questions and be honest if you don't know an answer. If that happens, offer to follow up when you know the answer.

5. Thank the legislator for his/her time.

6. Always follow up with an email referring to the conversation. This provides an opportunity to restate major points and provide any additional information [AONL, n.d.].

The nurse leader knows that relationship-building and interaction are essential to ensure that legislators truly understand how healthcare legislation impacts their constituents—individuals and at-risk populations who must access cost-effective, efficient services to ensure the best possible health and well-being. Legislative advocacy is a valuable skill that must be developed and used to achieve the success of the Quadruple Aim in healthcare. Nurse leaders must refine their advocacy skills to benefit healthcare recipients, their organizations, and their own colleagues. This is a challenge that they are suited to meet and accomplish.

As this book is published, a global pandemic confronts nurses and other healthcare team members who are on the frontlines of this crisis. Their heroism is demonstrated daily in caring for critical patients and supporting these patients' families while making difficult decisions to protect their own loved ones. No one can predict the future, but it is comforting to know that nurse leaders in all roles and positions partner in team-based care to meet current and future healthcare challenges impacting communities everywhere. This is truly Nightingale's triumph!

Afterword

No one can predict the future, but the author is certain that four aspects of this book will continue in the future.

1. Nightingale's influence will continue to be felt in nursing and healthcare.
2. Nurse leaders will lead healthcare initiatives locally, nationally, and globally.
3. The Quadruple Aim Framework will shape the direction of healthcare.
4. National and regional groups, like the Michigan Health Improvement Alliance (MiHIA), will foster positive changes in cost-effective care delivery for individuals and at-risk populations.

Appendix A.
Nurses' Influence Survey

Hello!

I am writing a new book about Florence Nightingale's influence in the practice of today's nurses to:

- Improve the patient care experience,
- Improve population health,
- Reduce costs, and
- Improve care team well-being (provider work life).

Nurses continue to be the most trusted healthcare profession and our influence in the evolving healthcare environment will be a major focus of my book. Your story is valuable in illustrating the success of nurses in achieving one or more of the above outcomes.

If you are interested in sharing your story with my readers, please respond to the following questions:

Demographics:

Name: (first name is acceptable)

Number of years in nursing:

Certified?   Yes   No   Number of certifications if applicable

Education (check all that apply)

ADN/Diploma   BSN   BS (other)   MSN   MS (other)

Doctorate in Nursing   Doctorate (other)

Nursing specialty:

Your story:

   1. What is your current position/role?

   2. Why did you become a nurse?

   3. What gives you the most satisfaction/pride in your current role?

   4. What is your most significant challenge/opportunity in your current role?

   5. What is your nursing philosophy (one sentence that describes how you feel about the nursing profession)?

   6. What is your most significant professional achievement and why?

   7. What advice do you have for future nurses?

   8. How do you care for yourself, so you can care for others?

   Any additional comments you'd like to share:

Appendix B.
Consent Information

Recently I sent you a survey requesting that you share your perceptions about your practice for my new book. You indicated that you would be willing to do this.

I think it is fair for me to describe how I plan to use these in the manuscript, so you can decide if you wish to be included in the publication.

I have attached a Synopsis showing how I plan to introduce each nurse leader to my readers using only your words about why you chose a nursing career. I am only using first names with no reference to any specific organization or location to maintain your privacy.

- A sample entry would be: "x has been a nurse for blank years and is currently a leader in a professional nursing organization. He/she has attained a PhD in nursing/healthcare and is certified in his/her specialty. He/she selected a nursing career because 'quote from your returned survey'"—first name only
- This will be followed by your nursing philosophy in your own words: Quote—x
- After the explanation about how these fit with the Quadruple Aim, I will devote a chapter to each of the 4 Aims and include quotes from nurse leaders' surveys that are applicable to the aim being discussed (improving the experience of care for individuals, improving the health of populations, reducing healthcare cost, and improvement of provider work life [team vitality]).
- Each entry will be a direct quote using only the person's first name. Each leader will *not* be quoted in each chapter.
- All of you will have shared how you care for yourself so that you can care for others, so I plan to include those direct quotes using only your first name in the chapter about the Fourth Aim.

- One chapter will include your advice for future nurses, again using direct quotes from the survey and only first names.

I will not use anyone's responses without permission. I am also willing to use a pseudonym if that is your wish.

After reading this, please tell me via email if you wish to be included under these parameters.

If so, please email your responses to me with your completed survey.

If you choose not to participate, I thank you for your consideration!

Best wishes!
Sue
Sue Johnson, PhD, RN-BC, NE-BC

References

Agarwal, P. (2019, April 22). *Timeline of Healthcare Reform in the USA*. Retrieved July 8, 2019, from Intelligent Economist: https://www.intelligenteconomist.com/healthcare-reform-pre-aca/

AHRQ. (2018). *Improving Primary Care Practice*. Retrieved September 24, 2018, from AHRQ: https://www.ahrq.gov/

AHRQ.gov. (2018). *5 Key Functions of the Medical Home*. Retrieved October 10, 2018, from PCMH Resource Center: https://pcmh.ahrq.gov/page/5-key-functions-medical-home

American Nurses Association. (2015). *Nursing: Scope and Standards of Practice* (3rd ed.). Silver Spring, MD: ANA.

ANA. (2015). *Code of ethics for nurses with interpretive statements* (2nd ed.). Silver Spring, MD: American Nurses Association.

ANA Enterprise. (n.d.). *Advocacy*. Retrieved September 22, 2019, from Nursingworld.org: https://www.nursingworld.org/practice-policy/advocacy/

ANA Enterprise. (2018, November). Healthy Nurse Healthy Nation Year One Highlights; 2017–2018. *American Nurse today*, 29–38.

ANPD. (2016). *Nursing Professional Development: Scope and Standards of Practice* (3rd ed.). (M. Harper, & P. Maloney, Eds.) Chicago, IL: Association for Nursing Professional Development.

AONL. (n.d.). *How to communicate with your legislators*. Retrieved September 22, 2019, from American Organization for Nursing Leadership: http://advocacy.aone.org/legislative-basics/how-communicate-and-build-relationship-your-legislators

APNA. (2019, Winter). *Nurse Leads Community Efforts to Reduce Youth Suicide*. Retrieved March 9, 2019, from www.apna.org: www.apna.org/suicideprevention

Associates in Process Improvement. (2018). *API-Associates in Process Improvement*. Retrieved August 13, 2018, from API-Associates in Process Improvement: http://www.apiweb.org/

Avalon, E., Washington, D., & Harris-Cater, G. (2017). Diversity: An integral concept in nursing professional development. In P. S. Dickerson (Ed.), *Core Curriculum for Nursing Professional Development* (5th ed., pp. 48–57). Chicago, IL: Association for Nursing Professional Development.

Batcheller, J., Zimmerman, D., Pappas, S., & Adams, J. (2017, June). Nursing's leadership role in addressing the Quadruple Aim. *Nurse Leader*, 203–206.

Beckett, C., & Melnyk, B. M. (2018). Evidence-based practice competencies and the new EBP-C credential: Keys to achieving the Quadruple aim in health care. *Worldviews on Evidence-Based Nursing, 15*(6), 412–413.

Berwick, D., Blanton, G., & Roessner, J. (1990). *Curing Health Care: New Strategies for Quality Improvement*. San Francisco, CA: Jossey-Bass, Inc.

Berwick, D., Nolan, T., & Whittington, J. (2008). The Triple Aim: Care, Health, and Cost. *Health Affairs, 27*(3), 759–769. Retrieved September 1, 2018

Block, I. (1969). *Neighbor to the world: The story of Lillian Wald.* New York, NY: Thomas Y. Crowell Company.

Bloom, S. L. (2010). Bridging the black hole of trauma: The evolutionary significance of the arts. *Psychotherapy and Politics International, 8*(3), 198–212.

BLS.gov. (n.d.). *Licensed Practical and Licensed Vocational Nurses.* Retrieved August 25, 2019, from U.S. Bureau of Labor Statistics: https://www.bls.gov/ooh/healthcare/licensed-practical-and-licensed-vocational-nurses.htm

Bodenheimer, T., & Sinsky, C. (2014). From Triple to Quadruple Aim: Care of the patient requires care of the provider. *Annals of Family Medicine, 12*(6), 573–576.

Boller, J. (2017). Nurse educators: Leading health care to the Quadruple Aim sweet spot. *Journal of Nursing Education, 56*(12), 707–708.

Breckinridge, M. (1952). *Wide neighborhoods: A story of the Frontier Nursing Service.* Louisville, KY: The University Press of Kentucky.

Butterworth, S., & Sharp, A. (2016, October 20). *Triple Aim framework: Why we should start with experience of care.* Retrieved September 2, 2018, from QConsultHealthCare.com Blog: http://www.qconsulthealthcare.com

Campaign for Action. (2019, January 14). *Racial/ethnic composition of the RN workforce in the U.S.* Retrieved September 9, 2019, from Campaign for Action: https://campaignforaction.org/resource/racialethnic-composition-rn-workforce-us/

Campbell, J. (2012). *In search of respect and equality: Life incidents of slave and free women in North American and Europe colonies.* Self-published.

CAPP. (2017). *What Every Candidate Should Know About Health Care.* Retrieved July 8, 2019, from accountablecaredoctors.org: http://accountablecaredoctors.org/wp-content/uploads/2017/08/capp_candidateprimer_2017.pdf

Carnegie, M. E. (1991). *The path we tread: Blacks in nursing 1854–1990* (2nd ed.). New York, NY: National League for Nursing Press.

Centers for Medicare & Medicaid Services. (2018). *HCAHPS: Patients' Perspectives of Care Survey.* Retrieved September 2, 2018, from CMS.gov: https://www.cms.gov/Medicare/Quality-Initiatives-Patient-Assessment-Instruments/HospitalQualityInits/HospitalHCAHPS.html

Chappell, K. (2016). The clinical learning environment. *The Journal of Nursing Administration, 46*(1), 1–3.

CMS.gov. (2018). *Value-Based Purchasing.* Retrieved September 5, 2018, from CMS.gov: https://www.cms.gov/Medicare/Quality-Initiatives-Patient-Assessment-Instruments/Value-Based-Programs/Value-Based-Programs.html

Coleman, M., McLean, A., Williams, L., & Hasan, K. (2017). Improvement in interprofessional student learning and patient outcomes. *Journal of Interprofessional Education & Practice, 8*, 28–33.

Cook, E. T. (1913a). *The Life of Florence Nightingale* (Vol. 1). London: Macmillan and Co., Ltd.

Cook, E. T. (1913b). *The Life of Florence Nightingale* (Vol. 2). London: Macmillan and Co., Ltd.

Crabtree, B., Nutting, P., Miller, W., Stange, K., Stewart, E., & Jaen, C. (2010). Summary of the National Demonstration Project and Recommendations for the Patient-Centered Medical Home. *Annals of Family Medicine, 8*(Supplement 1), s80-s90. Retrieved from www.annfammed.org

Darraj, S. (2005). *Mary Eliza Mahoney and the legacy of African-American nurses.* New York, NY: Chelsea House Publishers.

Davis, A. (1999). *Early black American leaders in nursing: Architects for integration and equality.* Sunbury, MA: Jones & Bartlett Publishers.

Doherty, Robert for the Medical Practice and Quality Qommittee of the American College of Physicians. (2015). *Assessing the Patient Care Implications of "Congierge" and Other Direct Patient Contracting Practices: A Policy Position Paper from the American College of Physicians.* Annals of Internal Medicine.

Donohue, M. P. (2011). *Nursing, the finest art: An illustrated history* (3rd ed.). Maryland Heights, Missouri: Mosby, Inc.

Dossey, B. M. (2000). *Florence Nightingale: mystic, visionary, healer.* Springhouse, Pennsylvania: Springhouse Corporation.

Emerson, R. W. (1803–1882). *65 Best Persistence Quotes and Sayings.* Retrieved from AskIdeas.com: https://www.askideas.com/65-best-persistence-quotes-and-sayings/all-great-successes-are-the-triumph-of-persistence-ralph-waldo-emerson/

Enders, T., Morin, A., & Pawlak, B. (2016). *Advancing healthcare transformation: A new era for academic nursing.* American Association of Colleges of Nursing.

Eskew, P., & Klink, K. (2015, November-December). Direct primary care: Practice distribution and cost across the nation. *The Journal of the American Board of FGamily Medicine, 28*(6), 793–801.

Feeley, D. (2017, November 28). *The Triple Aim or the Quadruple Aim? Four points to help set your strategy.* Retrieved August 16, 2018, from IHILine of Sight Blog: http://www.ihi.org/communities/blogs/the-triple-aim-or-the-quadruple-aim-four-points-to-help-set-your-strategy

Ferris, G., Davidson, S., & Perrewé, P. (2005). *Political skill at work: Impact on work effectiveness* (1st ed.). Mountain View, CA: Davies-Black Publishing.

Garcia Winner, M., & Crooke, P. (2011). *Social thinking at work: Why should I care?* Great Barrington, MA: The North River Press Publishing Company.

Godfrey, A. B. (1996). Quality Health Care. *Quality Digest.* Retrieved August 4, 2018, from https://www.qualitydigest.com/sep96/health.html

Health Literacy Universal Precautions Toolkit, 2nd Edition. (2015). Retrieved July 7, 2019, from AHRQ.gov: https://www.ahrq.gov/professionals/quality-patient-safety/quality-resources/tools/literacy-toolkit/healthlittoolkit2-tool5.html

Healthy People 2030 Framework. (2019, June 20). Retrieved June 5, 2019, from healthypeople.gov: https://www.healthypeople.gov/2020/About-Healthy-People/Development-Healthy-People-2030/Framework

Healthy People 2020. (n.d.). Retrieved June 22, 2019, from HealthyPeople.gov: https://www.healthypeople.gov/

Healthy People 2020. (2014). *Healthy People 2020 Leading Health Indicators: Progress Update Executive Summary.* Executive Summary. Retrieved June 22, 2019, from https://www.healthypeople.gov/sites/default/files/LHI-ProgressReport-ExecSum_0.pdf

HealthyPeople 2020. (n.d.). *Social Determinants of Health.* Retrieved July 8, 2019, from HealthyPeople.gov: https://www.healthypeople.gov/2020/topics-objectives/topic/social-determinants-of-health

Herbst, J., Raiford, J., Carry, M., Wilkes, A., Ellington, R., & Whittier, D. (2016, February 12). Adaptation and national dissemination of a brief, evidence-based, HIV prevention intervention for high-risk men who have sex with men. *MMWR Supplement, 65*(1), 42–50. Retrieved September 9, 2019, from https://www.cdc.gov/mmwr/ind2016_su.html

HHS.gov. (2018). *Strategic Plan FY 2018–2022.* Retrieved July 8, 2019, from HHS.gov: https://www.hhs.gov/about/strategic-plan/index.html

Hine, D. (1989). *Black women in white: Racial conflict and cooperation in the nursing profession 1890–1950.* Bloomington, IN: Indiana University Press.

Hine, D. (2004). Mabel Staupers. In S. Ware, & S. Braukman (Eds.), *Notable American Women* (pp. 611–612). Cambridge, MA: Belknap Press.

Houser, b., & Player, K. (2007). *Pivotal Moments in Nursing* (Vol. II). Indianapolis, IN: Sigma Thete Tau International.

Hume, L. (2018, December). An investment in staff well-being. *Nursing Management, 49*(12), 9–11.

Institute for Healthcare Improvement. (2018). *Improving Health and Health Care Worldwide*. Retrieved July 1, 2018, from Institute for Healthcare Improvement: http://www.ihi.org/

Institute of Medicine [IOM]. (2011). *The Future of Nursing: Leading Change, Advancing Health*. Washington, D.C.: National Academies Press.

IOM [Institute of Medicine]. (2011). *The Future of Nursing: Leading Change, Advancing Health*. Washington, D.C.: The National Academies Press.

Johnson, C. S. (2017). Ten steps to integrate nursing professional development in your organization. *Journal for Nurses in Professional Development, 33*(1), 40–41.

Joseph, D., Redwood, D., DeGroff, A., & Butler, E. (2016, February 12). Use of evidence-based interventions to address disparities in colorectal cancer screening. *MMWR Supplement, 65*(1), 21–27. Retrieved September 9, 2019, from https://www.cdc.gov/mmwr/ind2016_su.html

Judd, D., Sitzman, K., & Davis, J. (2010). *A history of American nursing: Trends and eras*. Sudbury, MA: Jones and Bartlett Publishers.

Kester, K., & Wei, h. (2018, June). Building nurse resilience. *Nursing Management, 49*(6), 42–45.

Knutson, L. (2019, June). Inside the nurse coach role. *American Nurse today, 14*(6), 37–39.

Koch, H. (1951). *Militant Angel*. New York, NY: Macmillan.

Kravitz, R., & Feldman, M. (2017, February 27). Reinventing primary care: Embracing change, preserving health. *Journal of General Internal Medicine*, 369–370.

Kurbo.com. (n.d.). *Healthy Habits Formed with Kurbo*. Retrieved July 5, 2019, from Kurbo.com: https://kurbo.com/

leapfroggroup.org. (n.d.). *Raising the bar for safer health care*. Retrieved June 23, 2019, from The LeapFrog Group: https://www.leapfroggroup.org/

Lewis, V., Colla, C., Tierney, K., Van Citters, A., Fisher, E., & Meara, E. (2014). Few ACOs pursue innovative models that integrate care for mental illness and substance abuse with primary care. *Health Affairs, 33*(10), 1808–1816. Retrieved September 24, 2018

Lewis, V., Tierney, K., Colla, C., & Shortell, S. (2017). The new frontier of strategic alliances in health care: New partnerships under accountable care organizations. *Social Science & Medicine, 190*, 1–10.

Li, Y., Kong, N., Lawley, M., Weiss, L., & Pagan, J. (2015). Advancing the use of evidence-based decision-making in local health departments with systems science methodologies. *American Journal of Public Health, 105*(Supplement 2), S217-S222. Retrieved Sepmmeber 22, 2019, from https://ajph.aphapublications.org/doi/pdf/10.2105/AJPH.2014.302077

Ma, Y., May, N., Knotts, C., & Devito Dabbs, A. (2018, March-April). Opportunities for nurses to lead quality efforts under MACRA. *Nursing Economics, 36*(2), 97–101.

Marshall, H. E. (1972). *Mary Adelaide Nutting: Pioneer of modern nursing*. Baltimore, MD: Johns Hopkins University Press.

Massachusetts General Hospital and the Massachusetts General Hospital Nurses' Alumnae Association. (2011). *Massachusetts General Hospital Nursing at Two Hundred*. (G. W. Pierce, & M. Ditomassi, Eds.) Boston, MA: Jeanette Ives Erickson, RN, MS, FAAN.

Massetti, G., & David-Ferdon, C. (2016, February 12). Preventing violence among high-risk youth and communities with economic, policy, and structural strategies. *MMWR Supplement, 65*(1), 57–60. Retrieved September 9, 2019, from https://www.cdc.gov/mmwr/ind2016_su.html

Medicaid.gov. (2018). *Managed Care.* Retrieved September 5, 2018, from Medicaid. gov: https://www.medicaid.gov/medicaid/managed-care/index.html

Melnyk, B. M., Gallagher-Ford, L., Long, L. E., & Fineout-Overholt, E. (2014). The establishment of evidence-based practic e competencies for practicing registered nurses and advanced practice nurses in real-world clinical settings: Prtoficiencies to improve healthcare quality, reliability, patient outcomes, and costs. *Worldviews on Evidence-Based Nursing, 11*(1), 5–15.

Michigan Health Improvement Alliance. (n.d.). Retrieved June 16, 2019, from MiHIA. org: https://mihia.org/

Michigan Health Improvement Alliance. (2019). *Dashboard 4.0.* Retrieved June 21, 2019, from MiHIA.org: http://dashboard.mihia.org/tiles/index/ display?alias=populationhealth

MiHIA/GLBRA. (2019, March). *THRIVE FAQs.* Retrieved July 7, 2019, from MiHIA. org: https://mihia.org/index.php/health-and-economic-initiative

MiHIA, GLBRA, & ReThink Health. (2019). *Stepping Out: Launching the First Stage of Interventions to Transform a Regional System for Health and Well-being.* Portfolio Testing. Retrieved August 25, 2019, from https://mihia.org/thrive-2/

MiHIA.org. (2018). *2018 Annual Impact Report.* Retrieved June 22, 2019, from https://mihia.org/index.php/about-mihia/impact-reports

Miracle, V. (2009). National Nurses Week and the Nightingale Pledge. *Dimensions of Critical Care Nursing, 28*(3), 145–146.

Mosley, M. (2004). Estelle Massey Riddle Osborne. In S. Ware, & S. Braukman (Eds.), *Notable American Women* (pp. 491–493). Cambridge, MA: Belknap Press.

Murphy, T., Denniston, M., Hill, H., McDonald, M., Klevens, M., Elam-Evans, L.,. .. Ward, J. (2016, February 12). Progress toward eliminating Hepatitis A Disease in the United States. *MMWR Supplement, 65*(1), 29–41. Retrieved September 9, 2019, from https://www.cdc.gov/mmwr/ind2016_su.html

National Academies of Sciences, Engineering, and Medicine. (2016). *Assessing Progress on the Institute of Medicine Report: The Future of Nursing.* Washington, D.C.: The National Academies Press.

National Nurses United. (2018, December 20). *Once again nurses top Gallup Poll as most trusted profession 17 years running.* Retrieved January 27, 2019, from National Nurses United: https://www.nationalnursesunited.org

National Quality Forum. (n.d.). Retrieved June 10, 2019, from Qualityforum.org: https://www.qualityforum.org/

National Quality Forum. (2014). *Multistakeholder Input on a National Priority: Improving Population Health by Working with Communities-Action Guide 1.0.* Retrieved June 15, 2019, from https://www.qualityforum.org/Publications/2014/07/ improving_pop_health_guide-1.aspx

Nightingale, F. (1992). *Notes on nursing: What it is and what it is not (Commemorative Edition).* Philadelphia, PA: J. B. Lippincott Company.

NINR. (2016). *The NINR Strategic Plan.* National Institutes of Health, National Institute of Nursing Research. Bethesda, MD: NIH. Retrieved September 2, 2019, from https://www.ninr.nih.gov/

NursingSchool.org. (n.d.). *Associates Degree in Nursing: Popular Fast-Track to a Solid Career.* Retrieved August 25, 2019, from NursingSchool.org: https://www. nursingschool.org/nursing-programs/program-types/associates/#context/api/ listings/prefilter

NursingSchoolPrograms.com. (n.d.). *The Nursing Diploma: The "old-School" Way to*

Becoming an RN. Retrieved August 25, 2019, from NursingSchoolPrograms.com: http://nursingschoolprograms.com/nursing-diploma/nursing-diploma/

ObamaCareFacts.com. (2018, November 16). *Health Care Reform Timeline*. Retrieved July 8, 2019, from OBAMACARE FACTS: https://obamacarefacts.com/health-care-reform-timeline/

Opperman, C., Bowling, J., Harper, M., Liebig, D., & Johnson, C. S. (2016). Measuring return on investment for professional development actiovities: Implications for practice. *Journal for Nurses in Professional Development, 32*(4), 176–184.

Penque, S. (2019, May). Mindfulness to promote nurses' well-being. *Nursing Management, 50*(5), 38–44.

Perlo, J., Balik, B., Swensen, S., Kabcenell, A., Landsman, J., & Feeley, D. (2017). *IHI Framework for Improving Joy in Work*. IHI. Cambridge, MA: Institute for Healthcare Improvement. Retrieved October 10, 2018, from ihi.org

Phillips-Jones, C. (2018, April 6). *Accountable care organizations and the Impact on care management*. Retrieved October 4, 2018, from CMSA Today: https://www.cmsatoday.com/2018/04/06

Pittman, P. (2019, July). Rising to the challenge: Re-Embracing the Wald Model of Nursing. *AJN,* 46–52.

Race and Ethnicity in the United States. (2018, September 4). Retrieved September 9, 2019, from Statistical Atlas: https://statisticalatlas.com/United-States/Race-and-Ethnicity#overview

Rhodes, S., Leichliter, J., Sun, C., & Bloom, F. (2016, February 12). the HoMBReS and HoMBReS poe un cambio interventions to reduce HIV disparities among immigrant Hispanic/Latino men. *MMWR Supplement, 65*(1), 51–56. Retrieved September 9, 2019, from https://www.cdc.gov/mmwr/ind2016_su.html

Satterfield, D., DeBruyn, L., Santos, M., Alonzo, L., & Frank, M. (2016, February 12). Health promotion and diabetes prevention in American Indian and Alaska Native communities. *MMWR Supplement, 65*(1), 4–10. Retrieved September 9, 2019, from https://www.cdc.gov/mmwr/ind2016_su.html

Selanders, L. C. (2005). Nightingale's foundational philosophy of nursing. In *Florence Nightingale today: Healing, leadership, global action* (pp. 65–79). Silver Spring, MD: Nursesbooks.org.

Sherman, R. (2017, June). The Leader Coach. *Nurse Leader,* 154–155.

Sinsky, C., Willard-Grace, R., Schutzbank, A., Sinsky, T., Margolius, D., & Bodenheimer, T. (2013). In search of joy in practice: A report of 23 high-functioning primary care practices. *Annals of Family Medicine, 11*(3), 272–278.

U.S. Congress. (n.d.). *The legislative process: Introduction and referral of bills*. Retrieved September 21, 2019, from Congress.gov: https://www.congress.gov/legislative-process/introduction-and-referral-of-bills

USLegal. (n.d.). *Legislative Process*. Retrieved September 21, 2019, from USLegal: https://system.uslegal.com/congress/legislative-process/

Valimaki, T., Partanen, P., & Haggman-Laitila, A. (2018). An integrative review of interventions for enhancing leadership in the implementation of evidence-based nursing. *Worldviews on Evidence-Based Nursing, 15*(6), 424–431.

vumc.org. (n.d.). *Faculty & Staff Health and Wellness*. Retrieved July 14, 2019, from vumc.org/: https://www.vumc.org/health-wellness/

Whittington, J., Nolan, K., Lewis, N., & Torres, T. (2015). Pursuing the Triple Aim: The first 7 years. *The Milbank Quarterly, 93*(2), 263–300.

Wilkie, K., & Moseley, E. (1969). *Frontier Nurse: Mary Breckinridge*. New York, NY: Julian Messner.

Williams, B. (1948). *Lillian Wald: Angel of Henry Street*. New York, NY: Julian Messner.

Wilson, N., & Leavens, A. (2015). *NQF/HHS Population Health Framework Project: Overview.* National Quality Forum. Retrieved June 10, 2019, from http://www.astho.org/PCPH-Collaborative/All-Partners/NQF-Population-Health-Framework-Project/5-19-15/

Woods, E., Bhaumik, U., Sommer, S., Chan, E., Tsopelas, L., Fleegler, E., Dulin, R. (2016, February 12). Community asthma initiative to improve health outcomes and reduce disparities among children with asthma. *MMWR Supplement, 65*(1), 11–20. Retrieved September 9, 2019, from https://www.cdc.gov/mmwr/ind2016_su.html

World Health Organization. (2018). *Diabetes Mellitus Fact Sheet.* Retrieved November 15, 2018, from WHO/Diabetes Mellitus: http://www.who.int/mediacentre/factsheets/fs138/en/

Yost, E. (1955). *American women of nursing* (rev. ed.). New York, NY: G.P. Putnam's Sons.

Index